I0489136

CHAOS IN MEDICINE™ SERIES

Volume 2

Healthcare for All:
Old Remedies and
The New Dispensation

By Nathaniel W. Wilson

INTERNATIONAL MEDICAL RESEARCHER

FIRST EDITION

Cover design: Tea De Santis
Illustrations: Tea De Santis
Layout and typography: Nathaniel William Wilson

Cataloging-in-Publishing Data

Wilson, Nathaniel William, 1976-

(published in the series, Chaos in Medicine™)
Volume 2 - Healthcare for All:
Old Remedies and The New Dispensation
ISBN-13: 978-1494808396
ISBN-10: 1494808390

electronically self-published through

Createspace
www.createspace.com

(an Amazon company)

paperback editions available through
www.amazon.com

Healthcare for All:

Old Remedies
and
The New Dispensation

to

Tea De Santis

L'AMORE DELLA MIA VITA

*for helping to build a nest
where before I filipendulously roamed about*

TABLE OF CONTENTS

Preface: SUMMARY OF VOLUME 1

(Sectional Synopsis)

Author's Preface
Sketches the author's context and details of the work environment that gave rise to the Chaos in Medicine™ Series of Publications, it also explains how the idea came about to name the specific case of ignorance "Obama's Blindness", mainly drawing from an indirect observation of Obama's movements around the world while still a US Senator in search of answers to a politically defined subset of questions pertaining to healthcare. The preface lays the foundation for understanding the seriousness of the problem as identified through official high-level medical services research, and sets the scene for a worldwide debate about the main reasons for failing healthcare systems.

Introduction
Explains the motivations behind writing the academic article which underpins the essence of this book series.

Abstract
Displays the abstract as it can be found in the academic article, as published in the *Global Journal of Health Science* (GJHS), volume 4, issue 6, page 1.

First Principles (Chapter 1)
This chapter is an adapted version of the entire academic article, but for a wider readership outside the normal confines of mainstream medical literature. It provides an extensive elucidation of the author's understanding of medical professionalism, medical sociology, the socio-religious basis of medical superiority, social class-based hierarchies in public healthcare settings, accreditation of medical degrees together with a renewed scheme for an integrated holistic healthcare educations framework, and objectives geared toward achieving more appropriate levels of integration and cooperation between healthcare authorities and organizations across the globe. The chapter ends with an in-depth explanation of "Obama's Blindness" and "The Missing Link in Healthcare" as two related yet distinct symptoms of a deeply set ignorance by which the medical profession was able to medicalize society to the point of today's huge (and growing) base of ineffectively-operated healthcare platforms.

Second Opinions (Chapter 2)
Starting with a description of a major botheration caused by the existence of a second opinion market and a general neglect for the importance of the first encounter with patients, this chapter focuses on the decreasing trend of proper patient examinations and the vibrant prevalence of situations involving non-effective referrals that could have been avoided. If patient examinations were done by not rejecting traditional philosophies involving exhaustive question-and-answer sessions (i.e. getting as much information from patients and eliciting detailed questions that could minimize patient visitations or lead to more accurate diagnoses after the initial contact between

2

healthcare professionals and patients), our prognoses for health would arguably be more progressive. The aspect of technology in diagnostic evaluations is considered, and also makes reference to the assumed general expectation that technological gadgets in the consultation room are always better and more effective. In the end, the argument moves in the direction of questioning the perpetual existence of a vibrant market of second opinions that does not necessarily yield either better outcomes for patient care, or the expected concomitant increase in indicators of basic health, or even a decrease in prevalence of chronic diseases.

Third Effects (Chapter 3)
In line with the idea of the butterfly effect, this chapter poses to the reader a question regarding the level of awareness of effects borne during medicalizing of society, effects on individual lives within communities around the globe. A shattering collage of impressions is sketched, also drawing from relevant personal experience, and the focus returns to the medical professional as the agent who needs to become more aware of the effects they create, even unknowingly, for these effects have significant consequences most professionals would never come to know about. This resulting enquiry calls on the proactive reader (more than the professional) to rise to higher levels of awareness about the effects of badly practiced medicine.

Fourth Reich (Chapter 4)
In this concluding chapter (of Volume 1), the medical profession is likened to a cult with an empire-like rule *over* the occupational world (globally). This is set off against the idea that the globalizing world is moving away from elitist mindsets; elitism has shown to throw the world into its darkest times; now, in 2013, as we usher into a new dispensation, the author calls for the abolishment of such elitist establishments with more equalized social constructs and mechanisms within the occupational world. Currently, medical doctors enjoy idol status in workplace environments where they can easily override decisions from other healthcare professionals even if these contributions from so-called *lower-rank* professionals could or would have led to better healthcare outcomes. The entire healthcare setting is structured around the elitist standing of medical professionals, seen from the holistic healthcare point of view, and it is this elitist structuring that must give way to more progressive attempts at making healthcare more affordable and effective.

***

At the conclusion of Volume 1 we have thus arrived at the height of criticizing the medical profession, from the point of view concerning status of medical professional in respective social and professional communities. However, as the projectile trajectory of an object in nature will obey the laws of gravity, we shall henceforth levitate toward a more pragmatic appraisal of the status quo within our healthcare environments. It should appear to the reader, at first, that the medical profession, itself, is likened to a cult, an oppressive minority who controls a subjugated majority; and that many of the major benefits within the collective healthcare framework practically goes virtually unchecked to those who could afford the steep university fees and lifestyles associated with medical doctors and their peers. It sadly even includes those who innocently and honestly managed to beat the odds of moving up the social class ladder by virtue of excellent academic performance only to eventually become as elitist-minded as many others already within the cultural mindset of the dominant culture thus represented. In exchange for having the privilege of becoming medical doctors, for having the respect and dignity that not many other people enjoy across a wide range of other professions, the crux of this inquiry is in the form of a simple question, *"what exactly have medical doctors been giving society over the last, say, sixty years that undoubtedly warrant their high levels of success in modern society?"*

This is the question that needs thorough contemplation, to the level of raising us to the awareness that we cannot continue to accept what has been handed down to us by falsely ennobled professionals without the equally ennobled measure of accountability that we as global citizens are entitled to receive. The question is exactly as we fear, *"Are we supporting a cult-type of profession at the expense of our (own) health?"*, and if we're indeed guilty of this supportive behavior toward medical dominance, why do we continue doing it; does it bother us at all? Saying that the medical profession is like a cult, or that it is indeed a cult, can be viewed as a very provocative statement; however, from our social health point of view, we choose to see it as a strategy in a humble troubleshooting mechanism – this would be the first question from a long list that serves to unblock many layers of understanding with regards to what we're actually dealing with when we talk about 'the main problems in contemporary medicine'.

Here we have arrived at the point of realizing that we need more practical answers to this question, or questions such as these; we need to allow ourselves access to the very mundane, routine issues of everyday medicine, those issues that directly affect people in and around the healthcare environment. Of course, the gateway-question, as we shall now call it, opens the contemplative mind to a host of other possibilities, and for this endeavor we need to prepare ourselves in adequate measure. It would be perfect if we would find pragmatic answers to each of the burning questions, but it also would be foolish to expect that all answers will have adequate pragmatic answers; therefore we need to select those questions that can provide us with more immediate, practical clues into the immediate future.

The answer to the question of whether the medical profession qualifies to be classified as a *cult* is not easy to formulate. Cult implies a religion, and religion implies a doctrine with (sometimes blinded) leaders and (almost always blind) followers. Declaring the existence of the "Fourth Reich", as was done in Chapter 4 of Volume 1, definitely alludes to the belief that a cult-like force is as work. However, before one announces the real existence of a proper cult, there must be tangible proof that followers are following a set protocol (doctrine) of action without much deviation from the beliefs and tenets of practice as set forth in organizational policies (scriptures), the transgression of which is punishable by (scriptural) law. Additionally, there are very strict criteria for kinship (membership) to this cult; only after thorough testing of studious followers' behavior (professionalism and academic fortitude) does the member receive benefits that far outweigh the initial investment, including peace of mind, financial security and protection from the enemy that seeks to destroy the kingdom. A bigger problem exists in actually proving that private, cult-like meetings are held, and that members of the cult are sworn in to defend the cause until death. Unions for medical doctors come into question, and a reminder is cast to the many secret fraternity-based organizations known for promoting the cause of medical professionalism amidst the changing global economic climate, ensuring a better, more progressive advancement for those very competitive individuals while the weaker ones are cast out 'into the wild', thus weakening the motivation toward better medical practice on the part of those who *didn't make the cut*. Proper cult members also transform the cult world into their entire dome of existence; those not considered worthy are forever placed at the perimeters, including those relatives and very close acquaintances with whom life is supposedly shared.

From a practical point of view, thus, it seems that we indeed have the type of situation onto which a cult-template can be fitted; it may be too early to officially label the medical profession with cult-like status, but with a somewhat deeper contemplation it does appear that there are many cult-like behaviors, practices and policies that underlie most of the everyday business that happen in the medical kingdom. Now, considering it all, it seems entirely justified to attach the word *pseudo-cult* to the medical profession; and for those in the profession but not part of the cult-like establishment, this may be challenging to admit, but the similarities are there, definitely, and its practical manifestations are not too deeply hidden, especially from a professional point of view; it is better hidden from the general populace, for obvious reasons. It stands to reason, therefore, that our healthcare environments are subjected to a cult-like operational mindset that seeks to alienate the benefits of the pseudo-cult profession towards members only, without the adequate consideration for the public at large in whose service they were placed by very trusting governments and politicians.

In candidacy for placement as a second-most important practical question, is the issue of distinguishing between those who practice medicine for medicine's sake and those who unashamedly ascribe to the cult-like dominion of medicine over the social-professional world. Here we have a tantalizing conundrum, one that perplexes the mind to a standstill worth noting. When we walk into a healthcare setting, how do we know we are dealing a real doctor as opposed to dealing with a *pseudo*-doctor? Is there a specific character profile that will help us, or are there other more subtle behavior manifestations that we can spot-check in our quest to make the very important distinction? (A loose definition: a real doctor is the doctor who's serious enough about medicine to take you very seriously, thereby dealing with you in the quickest time possible to help you find a way out of your medical predicament; the pseudo-doctor views you as a business client capable of generating more positive cash flow, and keeps you coming back for more ineffective treatments, or easily discards you upon the realization that you and your sickness will not be as economically viable, and also therefore not worth all the effort).

Do we have a *bad doctor* radar, or a *good doctor* detector that can reliably inform us on who to choose as our healthcare agents; in addition, if we have already been using these devices, how often were we rewarded with success of a good choice? How do we know that our doctors are those kinds of professionals upon whom we can always rely? I am sure most people have been exposed to this question at one point or another over the course of a lifetime and that this issue has the potential of ruining a day, a week or even the remainder of a human life. For some, sadly, this realization has never dawned; they have had the misfortune of inheriting the ill consequences of a bad doctor choice. Nevertheless, to return to the point of this paragraph, it is very difficult to distinguish between a good or bad doctor – in fact, I find it impossible despite my extensive observations and exhaustive psychological profiling.

In medical school, doctors are taught psychology (basic psychology, at least), like everyone else in most advanced degree courses, so they all know how to act the good role. It's at the order of the day to practice good behavior even if we don't mean it (it's a basic human imprint). Humans have always been good at acting, and the medical world, too, has its fair share of Oscar nominees. Therefore, from a practical point of view, the prospective patient should not be exposed to the situation of possibly encountering a bad doctor. A bad doctor can certainly shorten your life or end it – sometimes even good doctors do it, unintentionally, of course – but bad doctors do it more regularly, routinely. They even keep you on worthless medication for longer. It's always surprising that people will readily recognize the bad doctors on TV, but for some strange reason they cannot make similar, accurate judgments in their own lives when encountering the real-life medical situations. It's a matter of utmost significance and such importance that we cannot continue to expose ourselves to this tantalizing conundrum when we approach medical facilities. Because it so difficult to tell doctors apart, especially since one is so restricted when you want to exercise your choice of physicians in a medical facility, this volume seeks to underscore the urgency under which the corrective course of action should be taken – the medical authorities are at the brink of a massive change of approach to how medical doctors are accredited and absorbed into the medical structures within our respective societies. Since we cannot tell good doctors apart from the equally impressive bad ones, we would require the more proactive approach on the part of the medical educationalists and accreditation boards – hence the call for the overhaul of the medical qualifications framework, for the sake of rooting out the practice of bad medicine.

I definitely want more peace of mind when I visit the doctor. I want proof that my doctor (to correctly be called a medical professional) is actually better trained than other healthcare professionals on the street; there are many people who stopped visiting orthodox doctors but they seem so much healthier and in more control of their health, and more informed about it, too. If I am visiting a practitioner of traditional Chinese medicine, I do not want them to tell me that my orthodox family doctor doesn't know what's wrong with me, especially if the traditional medicine healed me immediately whereas the orthodox medicine had no effect on me. Indeed, this is a practical decision, but it also has economic consequences – the Chinese doctor charges me $50 including the medicine; the orthodox doctor wants $250, often excluding the medicine. In this case, my family doctor looks like the bad doctor – no self-respecting adult will refer friends or relatives to their own family doctors after encounters such as these.

In third place (possibly second) we have the question of doctors being overtly mobile and much less stable than before. Of what practical importance is this? Well, if you had the same doctor in your hospital or clinic for between five and ten years, your family would benefit more than when there's a new doctor every two years or possibly every year or semester? So then, why are doctors moving so much? *Bingo!!!* – the right question has been asked and we arrive at the heart of our argument: doctors are public servants, they deliver a crucial service to humanity – yet they are not frequently found in the places where they are most needed. As many of life's most difficult questions would have it, there are two very diverging arguments, but both remain very engaging because sound justifications on both sides of the divergent line are offered. Is it the doctor's responsibility to go where it is needed or is it the medical authority's responsibility to place the doctor where needed? Doctors are professionals and, of course, should have a choice of where they can work. On the other hand, however, if there's a medical professions authority that control how medical doctors are placed, then surely the doctors can be placed in more strategic locations, to maximize the reach of effective medical services. But can the authorities do this – do doctors go as requested? In most cases, probably not. The governments know this, but they cannot supersede the professional medical authorities. Or can they? Who is in control of whom, and what? We move in circles, because we cannot accurately place the locus of control. Or are there different loci of control? There are boundaries, i.e. regional, provincial, national and international – there are globalized organizations such as WFME and WHO – but how do we negotiate a restructuring of the medical framework to allow for a different mode of operation? We don't know. No one knows. But I think everybody involved here can admit that we have a serious problem that needs acknowledgment.

Acknowledgment would be the first step.

Acknowledgment would be the first mental step toward restructuring; then we would need feasible agreements as a follow-up practical step. The main practical difference between the practicing of medicine of today and tomorrow will be a visibly longer stay of doctors in the communities they opt for once they leave the training base. Why should doctors be so mobile when the healthcare settings from whence they're exiting are so poorly serviced, and the settings to which they flock so overtly serviced? Do we enjoy the great inequalities that exist? Some governments make huge profits when medical students are trained in their boundaries, but they lose as much (if not more) when the newly-qualified graduates are offered employment in other countries. Surely there must be more than just one other person who reasons that this situation is unacceptable.

So many students flock to the UK, Europe and the USA for training, never to return to their home bases, where they're needed most. Some do return, but against their will, due to contractual clauses. And strangely, most parents don't seem to care – as long as the son/daughter/husband/wife is earning good money elsewhere the family can live a good life. But what about the town, village or city left behind? In this way, developing countries will remain in the developing state, the developed countries will continue to gain more, and the world will continue in this poor state of healthcare inequality.

It is a long shot, but a shot worth taking; the answer lies in better, stricter, and more robustly enforced agreements between countries in the world with regards to movement of highly-skilled professionals. Some countries are offering citizenship in exchange for well-qualified individuals, leaving other countries at a loss; the better-developed countries offer much better basic conditions salaries but the results are the same: doctors are moving, too quickly, too easily, to locations with better financial prerogatives and incentives thereby crippling the very same healthcare environments responsible for their knowledge and expertise (in the form of training). Not only does the respective setting lose the multifaceted services of the professional, it also loses the momentum in service delivery gathered from all the time and effort of those other non-medical healthcare professionals. In many cases, the exiting medical professional is not replaced by a suitable replacement for a long time – sometimes even years. The problem is not difficult to comprehend, but the reader must certainly appreciate the complexity that comes with undoing a perpetual, collective action that's been allowed for many decades. The WHO admits that many of the new medical schools are "of dubious quality", which highlights the issue even more poignantly, but yet the inertia bounds us to humble acceptance, if not for the fear of change?! Something, somewhere, must yield.

A next issue for classification as a matter of high practical importance is the issue of medical technology. This is certainly a reality of everyday life; when asking professionals about this, this is *the* one, single area where we'd possibly have the most divided responses (of course, certainly worth investigative research efforts). When you really think about it, the advanced medical procedures are not always put in place because the general public demands it; many of the advanced equipment do not necessarily show its worth in terms of actually saving more lives than the times prior to invention of that specific novel technology. The medical profession oversees the main modes of medical research; medical research is dependent on the level of cooperation between doctors and the wider medical industry. Interestingly enough, the research that usually gets the expedited go-ahead from the masses of medical experts are those kinds of research that will translate itself into some tangible product on the consumerism market. This kind of thinking allows me to critically analyze the claims made by the medical profession, with the intention of actually establishing, very exactly, *what is meant when it is claimed that medical technology has changed our lives for the better*? Whose lives are better – the lives of patients, doctors, nurses, administrators, or even politicians?

In marginally few, select cases, calculated over the total number of medical patients in the world, it's a small percentage of people who effectively use the latest, most expensive medical equipment in ways that would not have been available through preexisting technology at that specific point in time. There is high competition for use of this equipment; mainly those with high levels of financial resources can use it. There are doctors who work exclusively for these highly selective patients, *selective* meaning *financially able*. But what about the majority of those alienated from use of the high-level expertise and equipment by virtue of not being able to afford these accesses? How do the claims of increased medical service standards and care apply to these more regular people, the category which include most lower through middle class citizens in the world? To regurgitate, these claims are that medical technology is responsible for the increases in effectiveness of medicine (or medical practice); that medical technology is changing the way in which medicine is practiced. These are big claims to make, especially if the medical profession cannot substantiate these claims with hard, epidemiology-based statistics on a more regular basis.

There is a different reality, however, in that there exists a certain type of *disconnectivity* on the street-level, perhaps a strong dissent for the so-called advanced (read: *expensive*) medicine that don't address the seemingly simpler health problems that are closer to the reality of most people. I can readily agree with the notion that technology has indeed led to increased prices and service fees for medical care that rely on the use of the expensive equipment, but it is hard-fetched to also automatically accept that the expertise also need to cost as much if the equipment is expensive. From the point of view of sound fiscal policy, there is not (or there should not be) an automatic increase in the service fees offered by the professional, even if the equipment used is expensive, and especially not if governments and some private companies subsidize much of equipment-related costs, including training. Where is the economic sense, then, if governments are claiming they're doing everything in their power to make medicine cheaper? The answer, of course, lies in the simple fact that maybe not everyone wants medical services to be cheaper.

Making medicine cheaper is akin to losing profit, something which the medical industry is not really willing to do. Can we allow the medical profession (and the dependent medical industry) to continue having their way? If you carefully think about it, the question can be rearranged toward a more progressive outlook: will the medical industry really lose so much if medical doctors were offered what they deserve, based on the idea that their earnings should be lowered to match those of equally adept professionals in the same healthcare setting? Some counter-intuitive extrapolation sees the rise of a new kind of medical market which could actually be as profitable, perhaps even more profitable, albeit for more people across a wider range of professions and businesses in the wider healthcare domain – the fat excesses of occupational dominance should thus become more evenly spread across the width and breadth of the working world. Better yet, such occupational dominance must be heavily reduced in an effort to completely annihilate the idea that medical professionals are the dominant role players in healthcare – they are strong players, but not the only significant players; certainly not always the most knowledgeable players. The idea is that more people could and should be trained to use the equipment; fees for the use of the expensive and advanced equipment can be absorbed into the subsidized costs by the hands of governments and huge private companies without having to resort to the remuneration that by, today's standards, are not justifiable by the mere laurels of the status titles of those who provide these vital medical services.

Basically, the expensive medical equipment, as it stands to reason, is not the main reason why medical doctors – especially the specialists and *super-doctors* – are so expensive. There are other reasons, reasons that may or not pertain to issues of healthcare, *per se*. The quality of this argument also depends on how we define occupational dominance, as well as how we justify the seniority and rank that doctors can enjoy in their workplaces relative to the host of healthcare personnel that surrounds them on a daily basis. The crux of this matter, from a pragmatic point of view, is that a leveling shift of authority (where status amongst healthcare professionals become more equalized) will be the one most basic, but very necessary step towards improving the intrinsic motivation amongst all other healthcare personnel and staff toward deliverance of a higher quality healthcare and service standard. If it is reasoned that the dominant status of doctors are well-correlated with the higher levels of knowledge and expertise they display, then we surely have to change the way in which the higher levels of knowledge are measured and accounted for in our healthcare settings. At this point, in 2012, the higher levels of knowledge on the part of doctors are not as clearly visible and are not as easily accounted for. Medical research that highlights this and other similar issues are either sparsely promoted or simply ignored by the masses of professionals to whom it is generally directed.

A number of other issues would comfortably fall within this category of pragmatic matters within healthcare that needs the most serious attention, but they do not, in my opinion, deserve higher priority than those mentioned above. For this reason, Volume 1 has come to an end but for the mention of one more point of practicality that might interest a handful of people, possibly some leadership figures within the general healthcare domain: what do I, as a medical researcher, stand to gain or lose by writing this book, and especially by the way in which I so outspokenly criticize the medical profession, medical doctors or the medical industry? Could I possibly also find myself in a conflict of interest? After all, I am a medical researcher whose success in life will ultimately depend on those who stand as ambassadors to the cause of making the world a healthier place. As an international medical researcher, social health researcher, medical sociologist, or whatever-other-name I might be described by, it is imperative that my main motivations are clearly understood, hence this dedication toward an explication of my social-professional context, for the mere sake of clarifying the base from which I extend my call for the complete overhaul of medical qualifications frameworks and changes of status-reward structures as we currently have in healthcare settings.

I know medicine, intimately. I know what it is supposed to do, I know what is does not do, I know what it says it wants to do, I know what it does that it is not supposed to do, I know what it keeps on saying what it says even if it does not do what it purports to do, and I know it's not always doing what it's supposed to do. I made it my personal business to study how the profession was able to keep on doing what it is doing today, how it was possible to block out or subdue any potential threats to its collective success and why it will continue to be difficult to change the course of the medical profession's voyage across the historic eras of humanity's occupational landscapes. Now, after a meaningful number of years, I understand why the profession does what it does. And in some instances, I dare say, you cannot hold responsible anyone in particular which is exactly why I chose to observe, as a third person, the interactions between the medical profession and its clients, or patients, so to speak – to better comprehend the situation and to describe what I could see, even if neither the client nor the professional were willing to fully acknowledge the situation they were in. The sick person acts the sick role and the medical professional acts the professional role. In this way, we all eventually benefit – or so it seemed.

At first, I guess, way back in the 1950s and 1960s, most people in the more exclusive neighborhoods (from the higher social classes) had access to doctors on a regular basis, in addition to some other social benefits. These people were outnumbered by the majorities of people from lower classes; doctors had easier schedules and customers they (the doctors) were happy to deal with. But now, in the 2000s, the era in which technology and society have changed too dramatically, many more people have access to doctors, giving rise to the undeniable situation that there are not enough doctors for all. Slavery and many other oppressive regimes have been abolished (even if not yet completely); governments are now expected to supply the same levels of medical care to much more people than what they could care to provide for in the past. I can see these things; I can see the effects of bad doctors, bad medicine, bad governments, bad fiscal policies; I see even worsened levels of service provision in other sectors of the human working world. I became a medical researcher, not by first choice – at first I enrolled to become a doctor myself – but I noticed the vicious effects and affects of innate human competitiveness, and saw first-hand how it impaired the ability of many qualified professionals to do what they supposedly aspired to do when they joined the vocational schools.

As a medical researcher, I want medicine and the practice of medicine, as a profession, to improve its healing effect on society. I am a medical researcher who really wants the medical environment to improve for the better. The quality of medical services delivery must improve, we need better medicines, we need better doctors and medical support staff, we need higher levels of motivation that would raise the standard of healthcare, and we need more people to become interested in increasing the healthcare profession's ability to provide better services and quality of workmanship. We need a society that will hold the profession more accountable, we need professionals who are better equipped to deliver the type of service that could lead to improved health conditions across the globe.

What would it mean to me? Why do I care? Well, it would be better for me too, if I were to stay a medical researcher; else I better change my stars, for then medicine (and the medical profession) becomes something more lethal than those other political campaigns that are currently dominating our world news by means of increased tension between people and nations. Instead of being accused of smuggling with nuclear weapons across borders of countries, the medical profession can be accused of smuggling with non-nuclear weapons of mass destruction: for example, blocking and controlling access to healthcare, leaving greater percentages of poorer people to die at the hands of plaguing health threats; increasing social tension between the rich (people who can afford to either become doctors or buy their expensive services) and poor (those who cannot afford it), thereby maintaining the demand for doctors to ensure their perpetual dominance in societies; using advances in technology to appropriate better working conditions for a select few while making it more difficult for those on the outside to gain access to what was previously called standard healthcare provisions. As a medical researcher I would like to continue to work in medical environments, alongside healthcare practitioners who also share the desire to improve conditions for all involved. I want my work to be respected just like anybody else would've wanted in any other occupational space – in fact, I would not be able to do my work if the majority of people in the healthcare setting would not agree with it. Researchers need permission from authorities; authorities, in turn, give permission when potential participants and institutions are acknowledged. It is prominently established that one's reasons for doing research are indeed toward the benefit of the respective society, in terms of improving health or the conditions under which healthcare is administered.

My main reason, then, for writing this book, is simply to raise awareness of a very big problem that is crippling our healthcare systems; by acknowledging it, we can collectively start to improve the conditions under which we receive our medical care. The public must develop more trust in the medical profession for being able to provide what they are paid to do: delivering a quality healthcare service at affordable costs. In the current mode of practice, there is no trust, barely any accountability except through damning court cases, and definitely no trustworthy mechanism whereby people from the lower to middle social classes can appropriate the necessary, basic levels of care that no human being on earth should be without.

I want money, of course. Of course I want to live a better life. Who does not? Of course I do not want to be poor. Who does? Ambition is the fuel by which a healthy soul can happily traverse the spaces of time, or, sadly so, it can be the congenital cataract in the eye of a blind person who will never see the beauty of a simple sunset. The money earned through a career in medicine can never be the main reason for studying medicine, for medicine, as we currently believe, stands as the paragon of healing occupations; as such it appeals to many of us as the most noble of occupations worthy of deep religious or spiritual appraisal. If increased status is easily achieved through acquisition of a medical degree, and if the increase in status becomes the all-important determinant in the individual's ability to be considered worthy of a greater salary, then we should surely halt the desperate attempts to wealth acquisition by means of a medical degree. Here I am willing to spend the remainder of my working years toward increasing the effectiveness of medicine; however, even as I have published papers that might raise an eyebrow or two, no university has offered me any substantial salary for my abilities to conduct proper research and publish high-impact papers, or even for getting doctors to be more cooperative with the other healthcare professionals. Yes, my work has been published and read by many, but because I am not a doctor, no public acknowledgment would come my way from those in my immediate working environment. Many doctors do not have time to improve their working conditions by means of ongoing research and quality control, yet they receive the recognition and increased salaries when things work better in their environments even if not personally performing any of the major work that ultimately led to better results.

My gut feeling is that something is not as it should be and if I could experience this type of feeling in my own workplace, then there would be others who might end up feeling exactly the same, especially when the recognition for their work was absorbed into the system that would ultimately shower the honors onto a more highly-placed colleague who, in fact, did not contribute much. My context is not difficult to comprehend: I studied at university, published a thesis and some papers, and dreamt of working for my government which in fact is in great need of high-caliber expertise. Being well-qualified, I expected a decent salary for the high level of work I can, and did, exhibit. To me, a salary of $99,999 p.a. would be enough – I could have a home, a car, once-a-year holiday, two children and a dog. On the other hand, the medical doctors are complaining when they receive $100,000 p.a. - and they go on strike when governments refused an increase. What do medical doctors need that kind of money for? And more importantly, people laugh when nurses and other allied healthcare practitioners are asking for a salary increase. Why should a director of nursing not receive the same as a doctor? Or why should young doctors receive more than nurses? The ideas within functionalism already described medical doctors as being no different than businessmen, and for this reason we must indeed stop healthcare from spiraling deeper into the abyss of dirty business.

The explication of my context is merely to assuage any fears that I would have private agendas under the table. It's a straightforward statement: something is wrong in the way medical doctors are allowed to be so ineffective while enjoying wealthy, lavish lifestyles and associated higher standards of living at the expense of dwindling healthcare systems and declining states of health – something needs to change, or as the movie title has it, *Something's gotta give*. My suggestion for the exact nature of change is based on observations as a medical researcher; furthermore, it is a notion developed from discussions with professionals in other fields, and there exists a general distaste for medical doctors who refuse to work with non-doctoral professionals from other fields based on the kind of attitude of "only talk to me when your qualifications are on the same level or better". It is a bold statement to make, but it is a realistic statement, not taken from a dream or concocted by wishful thinking. I could make an even bolder claim and say that the majority of the world's non-medical healthcare professionals, at current, readily agree with me; based on the results of many focus group discussions with medical students, nurses, doctors and patients. Many of the respondents within my focus group discussions specifically indicated that they would not admit these finding publicly, those admissions supposedly activated by a deep uneasiness with the subject matter – this, primarily, prompted further research which finally revealed even more startling revelations as discussed in the first chapter. I want to stay within medical research and I'd like to see, within my lifetime – should Providence will that onto me – how we can finally change the tide of healthcare toward becoming something more fortuitous to those who ride on it.

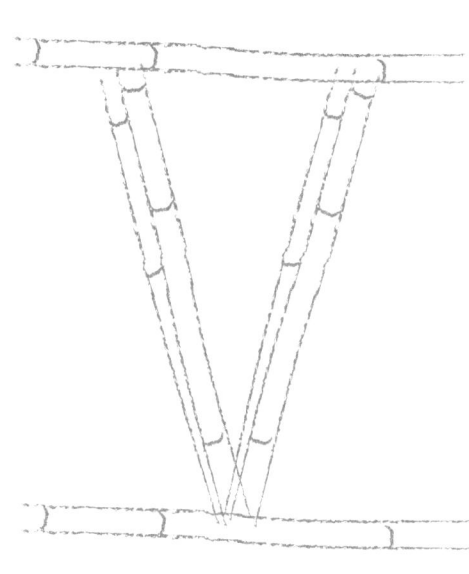

"Deep within the human constitution lie written laws of nature that should guide man in the conduct of his life."

Herbert M. Shelton

fifth LAW OF HEALING

Health begins at home, healthcare begins with you. A healthy home makes for healthier people. Healthier people make up healthier societies and healthy societies, in turn, make for a better, healthier world. Or, better said, this is the current "best practice model" of health. And to offset the chain reaction of health you don't need any substantial measure of wealth. You can be poor and healthy, or rich and sick – the choice about your health should not be linked to you economic state in life. Here I'm referring to those situations of health that fall under the category of basic, or as medical literature has coined it, primary health. It is unfortunate if you are very poor and cannot afford a specific type of surgery, but in that case we ask why your government and healthcare authorities cannot allow you to have that surgery. This is what Obama, essentially, is leaning towards, or what he should be getting at. In the matter of primary health, though, it is essential to realize that the majority of healthcare problems experienced by adults could have been prevented by a more serious approach to primary health during their childhood. I'm not saying children should be made experts on primary health; instead, what I am alluding to is the idea that we can teach our families, by starting at the earliest age, about ways of taking care of themselves that would prevent certain conditions from happening once adulthood is reached. Reaching the end of Volume 1, I began searching for answers to the question of how we could best approach a self-imposed change of healthcare habit. The *Fifth Law of Healing* appeared as a guiding light:

"there is naught but energy, for God is Life. Two energies meet in man, but other five are present. For each is to be found a central point of contact. The conflict of these energies with forces and of forces twixt themselves produces the bodily ills of man. The conflict of the first and second persists for ages until the mountain top is reached - the first great mountain top. The fight between the forces produces all disease, all ills and bodily pain which seek release in death. The two, the five and thus the seven, plus that which they produce, possess the secret. This is the fifth law of healing within the world of form." (From http://www.light-weaver.com/healing/toc.html)

Our religious differences set aside, there is one point that needs emphasizing, i.e. "the conflict of these energies with forces and of forces twixt themselves produce the bodily ills of man". Within the system of chapter titles for this series, the title "Fifth Law of Healing" was most appropriate (this is the fifth chapter, titled "Law of Healing"), but what must be understood is that I would firstly want to convey the sense of "Law of Healing", before arriving at a deeper understanding of the "Fifth Law of Healing" (as in the above quotation). It is philosophical to most, but for the few who already possess a more pragmatic understanding of this law, we know that by accepting ourselves as vessels of energy there is good sense in harnessing knowledge about how energies move within our bodies. When you read this, you are also in that world where "the conflict of the first and second [energies] persist for ages until the mountain top is reached". There is a law, and it states that we are sick because there are conflicts between difference forces of energy. It is a conflict within us, a natural conflict that we can learn about. Actually, it can be regarded as a natural-spiritual conflict, i.e. having origins in both natural and spiritual dimensions (if we regard life in two separate dimensions, of course). The other aspect of this law is that we will be sick as long as this conflict exists. Our (human) bodies are the seats for these conflicts and if we allow the right conditions to develop, then we'll be either sick or healthy, depending on the specific set of conditions at any specific point in time.

Collectively, as the human race, we are learning about how energy is moving through us. We do not know everything; it is not an exact science. Some will even say it is not a science at all. And at this stage most people still have major reasons for rejecting it – if it does not have a label as being a "proper science" then most people will not believe in it. And strangely, this is exactly why we have so much disease and ignorance in the world, and this is why we're not exactly as healthy as we'd love to be. The main issue, then, is that we tend to ignore things that seem impossible to grasp, and we never really bother with delving deeper than the initial layer of what seems to be impenetrable jargon of enlightenment junkies. Basically, we are afraid of being told that we know very little. This could seem like a small issue, but behold the state of health we have around us today! Our collective fears made it possible for better health to slip away from us; and if we cannot rise above ourselves then we'd never conquer any better states of wellness, no matter how much we spend on medicine and doctors. No doctor in the world is qualified enough to know more about our health than what we ourselves ought to know, and since this is something I believe with all my heart, I dedicate an entire chapter in this book to explain this extraordinarily simple claim.

We learn in school that our bodies have five senses; later we learn about the sixth sense, and then some other knowledgeable folk out there claim even more senses. Biologically, and scientifically verifiable, we are capable of at least five basic senses – seeing, hearing, touching, tasting and smelling. The sixth sense alludes to one's ability to sense other peoples' (or things') energies, so as to gauge good energy or bad energy. The other levels of sensations (in our ever-growing hierarchy of sensations) involves deeper spiritual states, of which we know little, of course, to judge by the current state of publications on the matter, also by the large number of public debates and disagreements about the legitimacy of claims surrounding human consciousness and the levels of our awareness regarding the spiritual world. Even if the world of spiritual enlightenment has also become a commercially viable domain for some, sadly so, we must not deviate from the main purpose in our collective quest to understand ourselves. Even if we do not know much about those other, deeper states of spirituality, we do know – and we must know – that our bodies are wonderful things.

Your body is a wonderful thing. It is a physical creation, capable of physical interaction with the universe made of other types of physical matter; but even more than that, it houses the core of what we are – our emotions, our spiritual beings. For this, we need to respect our bodies more, and we also need to pay attention to it more closely. It is my body and therefore I need to pay more attention to it than any other human being on this planet, even if they are the most superiorly qualified professional in the world. I am MOST AWARE of MY body, and I should be MOST AWARE of what MY body wants and what it needs. There is the simple truth: my body is my responsibility, and not that of anybody else. This could be our own law of healing, for the purposes of this chapter. My body will be sick if the forces of energy inside it is in conflict, and I am the only one who can proactively ensure that the counteracting forces are not constantly allowed to be in conflict – by simply removing the causes of conflict as soon as I become aware of their existence or their many different manifestations in my environment. Because your body is alive it becomes a vessel of energy. The only way to change that is to destroy your body and cause it to end its current form. Why don't we do that, why don't we kill ourselves? Well, is it because we really want to live?

When your body is busy perceiving (smelling, hearing, tasting, feeling, seeing), it interacts with the earth and the universe. Due to this interaction, and by means of it, energy is exchanged. And with so many different forces of energy out there, it is no wonder that these energetic interactions can lead to energy exchanges that overwhelm our bodily systems, hence disease. It's a word that literally could mean "not at ease". Either we get too much energy or too little of it. When it's not in the right proportions or the "most appropriate balance" of energies, then we'll not be very comfortable. With the information revolution having had its toll on us, we are in a better position to understand this "*dis*-ease". On the other hand, then, it makes perfect sense to try to understand how we can limit these unbalances of energies that impact on our bodies. Your body is actually your only real friend, and the one friend that will never leave you. One way to look out for your friend is through making some effort as to how best to serve it, to avoid the states of disease. There will be many diseases that you know nothing of, but if you pay attention really closely, your body would have showed you the way forward in terms of making some effort in addressing that problem. This is what doctors are trained to do, but from a more scientific basis. You, to the contrary, do not have to follow any specific scientific approach to understanding your body – you just have to learn to listen to it, or allow it to show you, or allow yourself to feel it more closely.

Once you enter this stage of awareness, you have started the real journey to better health. You are closer to your body than any other person in the world, so naturally you should know most about it. It is your duty, your first calling, your natural vocation, your ultimate responsibility, and your only best option to better health.

A funny thought came to mind – I shall have to write a separate book titled *"My body my best friend – the ultimate guide to a lifelong friendship with someone you can always trust"*. In essence, this is where this current discussion is heading – we need to know how to take care of ourselves. We humans have divided ourselves up into mental-psychological, spiritual-emotional, and physical parts. So, in order to take care of ourselves, we need to know the different parts of ourselves more acutely. Agreed – yes or no? Well, we may think that we know how to take care ourselves. I can see millions of nods, even hisses of sarcasm – who in the world does not know how to take care of him- or herself? So, if most people knew how to take care of themselves, why do we have so much disease, hunger, poverty and all these other vices? In fact, I did my own bit of hocus-pocus research by asking my friends if they knew how to take care of themselves. The answers were shocking. More shocking were some of the daily manifestations – how people dress, what they eat, their habits, and so forth. I could not share with them my real thoughts on the matter or else I would really only have one friend left in the world; what was most shocking was the simple fact that many adults had no idea about what foods are best suited for their body types, what clothes suited their body shapes most appropriately, and how often they were to take care of themselves by visiting doctors or dentists.

What is perhaps a strong claim to make is that most people have no idea of the realization that every day of living is a day for a medical check-up – not necessarily by a qualified doctor – but by you, in your own home, the environment in which you know yourself best. For most, medical issues only come to mind when the body lets you know of some minor or major disturbance that in some cases would already be too late to overturn back to a healthier condition. You are, in essence, your *own doctor* before you approach a medical doctor, and by opening yourself up to the idea you can possibly allow the notion that taking care of yourself involves some learning about your body – not as much as a doctor needs to learn in medical school – but just enough for you to know how to ensure a better, healthier quality of life without having to resort to always having economic problems when thousands of dollars need to be spent on hospital bills. Writing that book will be a good idea, but at this point it would better to stick to the topic at hand which is simply to gain a deeper understanding of our own roles in our health – and why we need to do something about it.

Your healthcare situation is not the doctor's responsibility. The doctor is trained to help you find out how to rid you of disease (if currently possible), he or she is trained to help you understand your responsibility toward your own health, but never in the history of mankind can they take responsibility for your healthcare, and you can never expect that of them, or demand it. It was never meant to be this way, not before, not now, and never in the future should it be that way.

Why so much emphasis on this simple topic? First of all, the topic is not as simple as it looks. Medical consumerism – the entire economic dynasty thereof – is dependent on people being very dependent on the medical services as provided by a secure medical industry. You and I are medical consumers. We consume the products of modern medicine and we are dependent on the services rendered. Some of these products and services are expensive – very expensive, in fact. It became too expensive for the majority of people who used to afford it before 2008, when the world experienced the glory days of lower inflation and huge medical bill payouts compared to the current state of affairs. As consumers, some of us become addicted – not being ready to admit it, though – and now we are very disgruntled by the idea that we cannot obtain what we used to receive when times *were better*. We start to say things, we feel different than what we felt before. We often feel undone, left out in the cold. We blame political party policies, politicians, federal or other governmental agencies. And once we start repeating some of these bad feelings and impressions it only takes a short while before we start believing it. We used to love our medical bills and the companies that gave us medical aid; we used to feel like we're riding the top of the world because we had jobs that paid these medical expenses (not in all cases, but for a relative majority of folk in the working class). Now, everything is different. After 2008, things changed, drastically, again. We did not know and there was no way we could know. So, how important is this topic of *being your own doctor*?

Well, for starters, if you were less dependent on your medical doctor and the healthcare services before the great global financial meltdown, then you would have felt a bit different about things than what you feel right now. If you were holistically-minded before, and your lifestyle actually already had the healthier habits as part of its daily itinerary, then you certainly would have felt different about doctors and nurses and the greater governmental plans for healthcare. The reason, today, for you being perplexed and disappointed, even annoyed, is simply that you were caught out; you were sleepy, not paying attention to the matters of your own health more closely, as you should have been since you were able to read and write. It is this course of action that we want to correct for; it is with the future in mind that we need to change how those born from us are guided into something better, something more rewarding. And this something, to give it a name, is called *individual health attentiveness* (IHA). It is possible that we can affect some changes even in our own lifetimes, provided we don't wait for another generation to be born before we finally decide that action is needed. If you are thirty years old today, then you will definitely see something substantially different by the time you turn fifty or sixty. But unfortunately, many people will read this, nod it off, not pay enough attention, and then we might have another economic meltdown, and people will actually start killing each other while standing in queues for medical equipment or service!

We need to increase our *individual health attentiveness*. Individual health attentiveness. **Individual health attentiveness**. **INDIVIDUAL HEALTH ATTENTIVENESS**. Say it a few more times. Emphasize the phrase. Whisper it, shout it, say it to a friend, call your mom or dad, and say it at the breakfast table before the family dispatches for fulfillment of their daily routines. One of my high school teachers used to say that the brain needs to 'hear' itself about ten times before it remembers something forever. Look up every synonym known for each of the three words. Write it all on a poster; project it onto the ceiling so that you can see it at night. Do something about it. Think carefully. What can I do to become more attentive about my health? Remember the

Law of Healing from the beginning of the chapter? Let's combine the two distinct concepts; let's merge them into one concept. Let's collectively create a simple law that will stand the test of our time:

Table 1 Individual-focused Law of Healing

Law of Healing	Individual Health Attentiveness (IHA)
"the conflict of these energies with forces and of forces twixt themselves produce the bodily ills of man"	"an individual's increased awareness about the exact state of his or her own health and knowledge on the maintenance of a healthy state of being that must serve to minimize the occurrence of trauma, disease and medical discomfort"
Our understanding	Our understanding
if we understand more of how the conflict between these energies can be minimized, we will have a healthier approach to life based on the knowledge so gained	in order to experience a better quality of life, regardless of personal economic state, our main responsibility is toward self; to firsthand inform ourselves with regards to maintaining a healthy state of mind and being; our actions to be regular and consistent, as with a very productive habit
The individual-focused law of healing (IFLoH)	
Every individual has the responsibility toward self to ascertain, to the best of available current knowledge, their exact state of health, by way of self-learning toward understanding of the interaction between their physical and mental bodies with respect to the immediate environment; to act on maintaining a healthy state of mind and body; to regularly seek official validation of health status, not only when mental or physical distress is experienced, but as a regular, consistent act of ascertaining health status for the sake of being informed; and to report abnormalities, if any, to those empowered (legitimate healthcare assistance)	

What would the purpose of this be? How does it allude to anything different from what has already been said or done? This is from a different point of view as the one used in Volume 1 of this series, but remember, it's from an individually-focused point of view. So, let's look at the role of the individual in his own life in terms of healthcare, taking into account our law of healing. The individual has the responsibility (read: *not* the doctor) to find out what is happening inside their bodies. It is not the doctors' responsibility to find out what is wrong with you. You have to find out what's wrong. Because it's your responsibility, you must make an effort to consult the doctor. You ask the doctor for help. The assistance and service thus provided will aid in your recovery, if recovery is possible. Basically, the doctor's responsibility is to provide a diagnosis, based on what you say about your situation. The doctor must do this, if he or she can, and within the shortest time possible. This is not always possible. It is still your responsibility to find out what's wrong inside your body. The doctor has a professional responsibility toward you but he or she does not have the personal or individualistic responsibility to perform this duty – it is your body, not the doctor's. There is a difference even if it may come as a shock.

This may sound absurd, but if you take time to study medical sociology then the well-known idea of the sick role has been clarified before and that people also come out to *act* the *sick role* with the doctor. It does add its fair share of complications to the doctor-patient relationship, but it is a phenomenon that occurs very frequently, frequently enough for it to have this behavior-based label in academic literature.

As a global population in dire need of more efficient service we also need to take cognizance of the fact that we cannot continue to act out the sick roles. Returning to the issue of finding out what your problem is, most people do not have the technical know-how for describing what's happening in the body. But that wouldn't be the purpose – you do not have to describe your problem to the highest degree of detail. Let's consider you in the guise of an experimental case study subject with a very typical problem. You have a pain in your right side, and it's been paining for a few days, almost a week. Your right side, just below the lowest rib cage bone, is possibly due to your liver having some kind of difficulty; finding out the cause of the pain can be helpful, for if you know you've not been drinking excessive levels of alcohol then it would be advisable to pay the doctor or nurse a visit just to check (assuming, of course, that consumers of excessive levels of alcohol try their best to stay away from any legit medical environment – by no means is this acceptable, but it's a fact of our daily lives). If, for whatever reason, you cannot go to the doctor, then asking around can also help. You may even have a developing case of appendicitis, so it would be responsible for you to help yourself, for the sake of your own health, to seek some care or assistance until you know what is causing that pain. Ignoring the pain leads to other problems – it has far-reaching implications for your family, especially if you're the provider and suddenly one day you cannot go to work because of that same pain returning, without any warning signs, with a more severe acuteness that actually prevents you from doing anything. By ignoring the pain, you display an act of being irresponsible. It is your familial situation that demands action on your part, but it is an even higher level of responsibility for yourself that should ultimately cause you to act. Better yet, if you're raising children by the time you're reading this, it will be a tremendous bit of education if you can tell them that you have an inherited liver abnormality – by the time they grow up, you would have told them about the symptoms and what to look out for to prevent any severe medical trauma from happening when it's far too late to do anything. The point here: it's not the doctor that needs to do this; it simply is you, and only you – not your mother, father, brother, sister, uncle, aunt, niece, cousin, nephew or any other relative or kin on the face of this earth.

You are your own, first-hand caregiver. You should give yourself some care. This brings us to the point of the preceding paragraph: we need to start taking care of ourselves – properly and decently – like we were taught to do when we were little, like when we took care of our younger siblings or our friends at school. This fact, alone, makes this statement, and our new law, relevant. Too many patients, from all around the world, seemed to have given up hope and care, and have subsequently left the responsibility of their health to someone else – a relative, a spouse, or even the doctor. If more people had collectively understood this individual-focused law of healing, then our prognoses would have been much improved.

With increased levels of IHA comes the issue of authority. Who has authority over your body? Don't be alarmed, but this issue of authority over your body is a hugely debated issue; and it is always under review due to many social, political, religious, ethnic and spiritual modalities that frequently make their way into legal battles between the medical professionals and patients. It's no small matter. The mere mention of the word *authority* will raise the mercury out of the tube in most medical settings. I must indeed state a disclaimer: I am not contesting authority over another individual's body, it is merely a discursive attempt, and I do not associate myself with any one established rule of life other than individualistic ownership as declared in the next sentence. As an adult of clear mind and conscience, I have authority over my own body. So, I will decide who gets to do what with my body, in terms of healthcare interventions and procedures. For you, it's your body and you have authority over it (for adults, of course, in most countries; for most minors, let's assume their legal guardians to have this kind of authority in matters pertaining to healthcare and medical procedures). If you have the prime responsibility to yourself in terms of healthcare provision, then the prime authority over your body must also reside with you, of course, unless you are legally declared unfit to accept authority. Am I stating the obvious? Well, not exactly. You see, the orthodox, westernized medical doctor is frequently under fire, for obvious reasons. They are required to do patient examinations. Some patients assert authority and some others do not. For the patients who do not assert authority over their bodies, do doctors and other healthcare professionals assume authority, coercing those patients into predetermined outcomes that superficially satisfy the requirement for immediate diagnoses and treatment? For the patients who assert authority by refusing certain basic examinations to be performed, can the doctor insist of being allowed those examinations even if it goes against the patient's initial expectation or allowances? Then, if the patient is not satisfied with the diagnoses of services offered, and it turns out that some erroneous conclusion was drawn due to a lack of observational validation caused by the asserted authority to refuse the examination, what becomes of the responsibility toward one-self for finding out what is wrong with you? I should perhaps not mention it here, but it is a well-known fact that people can easily achieve predetermined diagnoses from physicians without physicians having even lifted one sleeve of a sweater or without having to draw any blood on which to base a diagnoses. Patients are not always aware of the authority they can assert and they assume it is safe to leave it to the doctors to decide. Doctors, nurses and other healthcare professionals are sometimes not aware of the fact that patients have no idea of authoritative ownership and in this huge, gray area of uncertainty many mistakes are born; some patients yield all authority to the knowledgeable professional, and by this the knowledgeable professional often misses the real diagnoses due to the patient's complete unawareness of individual rights. Some doctors do not know that for some problems there is no other way to a diagnosis than through physical palpitations or taps; some patients do not know that doctors are afraid of touching them, for fear of litigation and other negative social responses. The world has changed, but the doctor-patient relationship has been left in the dark of yesteryear, and the silences surrounding both parties has changed the positive potential that once lay hidden in this very important relationship within the healthcare settings.

Even more distressing is the ownership of authority with regards to the history taking and initial patient examination in healthcare settings. This matter can be dealt with more elaborately in subsequent publications, but one aspect of the distress needs to be highlighted: the medical profession has taken complete ownership of the patient's first encounter with the medical setting, and for this reason the term "doctor-patient relationship" has been coined. Unfortunately this has alienated the patient from the other healthcare professionals in the setting, and this alienation, as it stands to reason, could be largely responsibility for the poor levels of service delivery to patients when doctors are not available at healthcare institutions. The patient needs to understand its authoritative role in respective healthcare situations, to the degree that each patient can comfortably assert the necessary authority with regards to different aspects of the holistic healthcare experience. It remains the responsibility of the medical profession to relinquish any claim on authority over the patient and diagnoses; the new dispensation of global health requires more integrative cooperation and the entire healthcare team needs to take collective responsibility for providing the patient with the appropriate levels of medical care and services. Gone should be the time that the medical doctor claims any superior authority on matters that concerns any patient and henceforth all healthcare provision should be undertaken in the mindset of integrated service provision or other modes of operation that will ensure more holistic approaches. It is of vital importance that patients are also educated to the degree of understanding their own roles in the medical jungles of misplaced authority.

It can be said that issues of authority could be linked to our consumerist mindsets. In any case, we probably don't need any lessons in consumerism or what consumerism has done to us. Do we also have to include the issue of our health in our contemplative analysis of how consumerism has wrapped us in its sheath of greed and clouded murkiness that prevent us from understanding how we've allowed ourselves to sink knee-deep into bottomless depths from which it seems impossible to escape? It is a difficult topic to raise and it's a difficult issue to face, especially when things are not going too well, from both health and economic points of view. For this very reason I appeal to the reader's best and clearest conscientiousness regarding the matter at hand; there is simply too much to lose by ignoring a strong warning that seeks to inform on how to change the status quo within our personal lives, a necessary change that will render us more independent on the public services and products without some of which we could have done without. Some laws of nature cannot be ignored no matter how much more knowledgeable we become; in fact, the more we discover the more we realize the wisdom in having inculcated the laws of nature into our everyday lives. Such is the case for the individual-focused law of healing: it is our prerogative to fend for ourselves, to protect those we love, to honor our physical bodies for the sake of an improved spiritual experience of life; to become independently aware of our roles in our health without having to develop any dependence on any drug, medical service or healthcare institution that seek to imprison us in our states of helplessness – a helplessness born by an apparent lack of knowledge, inferior self-esteems or even perceived states of despair due to poverty or other social vices. When we say "law of ...", a certain sense of authority is implied – what authority, in the case of healthcare, is the most powerful?

To illustrate conceptually, let's consider the statement: if everything with mass on Planet Earth is subjected to the Law of Universal Gravitation then every human being with a body on Planet Healthcare is subjected to the (Universal) Law of Healing. By whose authority is this law valid, and under what conditions must it be declared valid or deemed invalid? Well, if you believe that all energy is God or that God is all energy, then you accept that all energy obeys some kind of law regardless of the form of that energy. If you happen to be atheist, agnostic or some other kind of -*eist* or -*ian*, then you must surely have some appreciation for concepts such as gravity, you could even believe in it because it's proven to less abstract and more real – if you jump up, away from the floor, you will certainly return to the spot you jumped from without having to force yourself back there. We'd then all agree – some laws are to be obeyed even if you want to or not. By the same token, then, we accept the law of healing: something goes wrong somewhere, in terms of energy flow, and this misalignment of energy can cause disease. Disease is a manifestation of something that does not align very favorably and it will affect us if we allow the conditions for it to develop, whether our allowances for it are conscious or subconscious. Different diseases manifest in different environments, it affects different kinds of people differently, and it surely demands different types of responses based on a very wide range of factors – but there are a few things that all diseases do – firstly, they all indicate that something is wrong, somewhere, somehow; secondly, they demand serious attention; thirdly, they make us all have something in common, just as we're all subjected to gravity. The door is now opened to understanding how the issues of healthcare take such a center-stage position with respect to the things in our lives we deem most important. It is this knowledge, namely that our health is of central importance, that forms the essence of the vastness of the healthcare empire, which elevates the issues of authority and power in our lives to such an extent that we could never over-think the importance of this seemingly simple universal truth. Yes, there is a certain truth here; health and disease form two extreme manifestations of a very simple truth captured in a simple law. The truth about us being healthy or diseased relates to us being subjected to natural forces in our environment that obey the law of healing - whether or not we do it consciously.

Most often the most complex situations are unraveled with simple truths and this is something that will continue to baffle us. With our health and the related issues of healthcare it is no different. We sort-of already know what is right for us from a very early age. Do we follow our inner voices or do we allow our voices to be drowned out by the noise of contemporary society offering such easy advice and quick-fix solutions? No matter how advanced technology becomes, some basic things will always remain most effective, and most advanced, for that matter. Pumping your body full of steroids for the six-pack does not make you a healthy person, even if the photo of your six-pack is published in a glossy magazine. Still, after all the years, moderate running and walking still remains the best way to keep fit, as some mothers will tell you when taking the kids out to play for two hours every day. Your health is not a quick-fix issue; it does not belong under that categorization and should never have been subjected to the mass market consumerism where even the biggest losers (of fat) can become celebrities. Underneath all of this there's a law of healing, and true healing will only depend on how well you allow the energies around you to minimize the conflict in and around your body, your system, your temple, or whatever other name you want to give to the physical part by which you are known.

***

Laws of nature are not very difficult to obey unless your mind discards these laws for other seemingly better-dressed artificial laws that come in the form of popular press and media. If your mind if full of fancy clutter, you can easily miss the simplicity of how to keep healthy – from within and on the exterior. The book, *The Tangled Wing: Biological Constraints on the Human Spirit* (author Melvin Konner), was one of my earlier and most secure inspirations toward a deeper understanding the mind-body connect; it addresses this issue of how the body and mind are separate entities within the same body, or how they're the same entity with different manifestations (people have traditionally chosen a side, either mind-body separatists or body-mind unionists). A few lines into the soul of this insightful book does indeed pave the way toward a deeper appreciation for the natural laws which govern our lives by virtue of how they affect our bodies and how our bodies respond to the environment – regardless of our chosen religious or spiritual alignments. Another book, *Born to Run* (author Christopher McDougall), very eloquently portrays the resilience of the body in face of a very strong mind whose composition is based on inheritance of genetic material that predisposes a 'super-tribe' of people to almost unnatural levels of endurance and fitness. These are all clear indications that our bodies are such wonderful beings and that we should take better care of it. What, then, are we waiting for? Must something too dramatic happen first (such as a major economic crash, or a steep rise in drug addictions, or a fifty percent increase in medically diagnosed chronic conditions) or are we finally able to affect a global change, on a massive enough scale, to force a change in the hand that purports to feed us but has actually been getting fatter itself, off our tax money?

What concerns most is that the human spirit can endure lots of suffering, torture, pain and even outright annihilation – are these the outcomes we prefer? Have we given up, did we throw in the towel, are we ready to kick the bucket? Are we really satisfied with how things are, are we really as content as we'd want to make others believe? Well, the law of healing has been written and we best live up to it else we face even darker and gloomier times ahead.

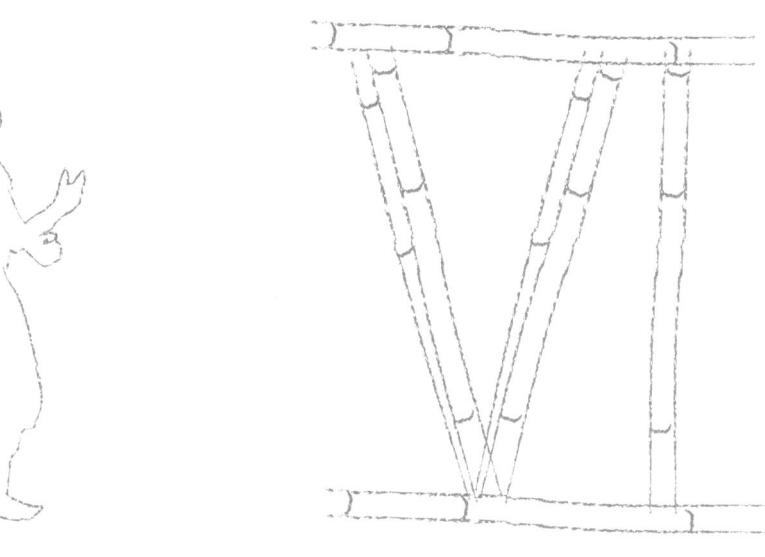

"Courage is being scared to death, but saddling up anyway."

John Wayne

sixth STEP

"What is the purpose of a journey was it not for the next step...? But what of the next step if there never was a first?"

How do we take the first step, and the next step forward? If we compare our journey to an activity involving climbing a ladder with an unknown number of steps, it is one feat to have arrived at yet another rung higher up, but now the knees need to be stronger and the arms steadier else we lose balance of all that were trifled over. At this point, the number of people to have opened up to the main idea of writing this book is only one, but the information herein could be transformed into action that could affect millions of lives. In the milieu of contemporary society one must indeed take a sizeable measure of the many diverging facets of an almost infinite variety of cultures and ways of living. We are all so different, yet we experience the same gravity, and this is precisely that motivational whisper that can usher us further toward a more progressive understanding of our collective plight. In both volumes of this series, thus far, this chapter would prove to be the most challenging. There is this fear that all comes to naught were one not able to convey a reliable forward-thinking approach that could guide initial steps for many people to whom the whole idea of "do-it-yourself (DIY) health improvement" is still too foreign, too cloudy, too impossible, or too grandiose; there exists a certain skepticism with regards to people who write and publish under the banners of being experts. Current collections of popular literature are filled with writings of those publicly endorsed as experts, but yet it is hard-pressed to find large enough numbers of people – who heed the advice of the experts toward an actual change of approach to life, or even in just one single change of behavior or action that could translate into a massive global change in the status quo of healthcare services provision and more organic individual approaches to health.

Human beings, generally, are resistant to change. Our souls yearn for the changes, but the flesh is much weaker. Writers know this, but often the motivation behind writing for the benefit of others involves many hours (sometimes days, weeks or even years) of doubt, denial and loathing self-criticism. In the literary world, as a result, there comes a certain (ethical) responsibility to stay true to the purposes with which you set out to write, which most times – during the process of writing – seem like the most impossible thing to achieve. Many writers will agree that as you write the preceding sentence, more doors of thought are opened up only after you see what you wrote before, and never at one stage would you exactly know what you were writing about until the end of last words have been placed. I am reminded of one of my favorite quotes by Blaise Pascal,

"Words arranged differently have different meanings, and meanings arranged differently have different effects".

So true that is, hence my procrastination over the last decade, but in the end the idea must be set free. It constantly revisited me; it made itself unbearable, even after my strongest objections and resistance. It must be given wings to fly the world in search of impressionable young minds hungry for those meanings that will impress significantly in generations to follow.

I do not claim to be the expert; I am knowledgeable about this issue, knowledgeable enough to share my very interesting observations, conclusions and ideas that were borne during this explorative journey. These ideas are worth sharing; I trust it is accepted in the spirit of sharing those things which are closest to your heart, for the sake of reaching out to a world in need a gentle reminder about how we cannot lose sight of our most precious gift on earth.

***

Alas, before we can take that step we need to assess where we are, or better, we need to assess where we're not. Before reading this book, did you by any chance read any other book with the same or similar type of message or idea? If so, how did that make you feel? If you felt very motivated and driven to action, did you do something about it in your own life? If not, did this volume of material make you feel anything different, something that might drive you to action? As you may imagine, there could be a million questions such as these in order to establish exactly where we stand in terms of coming to terms with the root or core of our healthcare realities. What we'd basically have to establish is whether or not we're ready for accepting something so simple that could help us change the world in a way it hasn't been changed in many, many years. I do not want to rely on analogies too much, but the story in the *Qur'an* or *The Bible* about Noah's Ark serves as an illumination. How could the people know that such a dreadful flood was indeed going to end their lives – Noah was said to be drunk and not as educated as some of the more prominent people of his time? The word 'flood', it is claimed, did not exist in most of the current conceptualizations of nature at the time – why on earth would people heed the advice of someone as lowly as this man who was afflicted with mental problems

54

so much so that he started building an ark, a massive project that served no purpose? In the same, how can we know for sure that our healthcare situations will get to such a point that it would almost be impossible to take care of yourself or your family in terms of providing frequent basic-level health?

Well, from a more contemporary understanding of the world, we have since developed a more scientific approach to life and scientists have made strides in terms of teaching us to extrapolate from our current positions into the future, based on currently available evidence that point to trends of events. It's not as if this type of extrapolation was not used before the dawn of our scientific mindsets – ever since the dawn of history (as we understand it today) there have always been some people known for "telling fortunes", "forecasting the future", "predicting the occurrence of natural events", "communicating with the dead as a means of seeing into the future", and so forth. What we have here, from our healthcare perspective, is a situation by which we can clearly see, through published evidence from all around the world, that our healthcare needs are not met adequately. We have major disparities in our societies, reflected in the many hierarchies in our homes, churches, workplaces and social groupings. Some people stand up against the rise of more disparities, others help to enforce it, there are many who simply don't care as long as they're not involved. Others, sadly, benefit from the disparities, by becoming wealthier, while those they pry upon are becoming weaker and poorer. I don't think we need a thesis on how bad these types of situations are – the news headlines are conveying these sentiments on an hourly basis – no matter where you go. I could easily claim that our (western-influenced) healthcare systems are in a state of chaos. And I need not be too concerned about the criticism on this single fact. It's similar to stating, "politicians are paid too much money for work they do not do". Most people will readily agree, in silence, but when pressed for publicly showing support, those agreements vanish into obscurity.

This, then, is where we stand. We have a big problem with healthcare, not only where we live or where we come from, but across the whole world where orthodox medicine has been allowed to state its claim on society. If we can agree on this, then we can start to take the first step toward healing ourselves of a most corruptible agent in our midst that is taking away our chances of living better lives. According to Newton, as his formulation of the laws of motion is still accepted after so many years, a force must consist of two components: an agent and a system. We are the system, the everyday people who need the services and products of the medical industry; the service provider is the agent – exerting a force on the system. If we understand our role as the system more clearly we should know that no force in life can exist without a counterforce. The agent has now wielded too much force onto the system; the system is cracking and needs to exert that force back onto the agent; we (the system) cannot continually absorb the punch of the agent without holding it accountable for the pressure exerted – sometimes on very unsuspecting members of the public who plainly just need a good service at more affordable costs.

We are thus not at the stage where we have to invent everything from scratch. We cannot level the buildings and cancel (governmental) state functions involved with healthcare. We don't have enough money and resources to build new medical schools everywhere

where we want them – as close to our homes as possible – but some governments are doing better in terms of providing some form of service in many regional districts in each town or city. Point is, the infrastructure of the current system is already there, it's set, and we'd better make best use of it, but we cannot infinitely continue to protest and strike to the point where normal disruptions of service now become the norm, as opposed to normal functioning hospitals and clinics that become the exception to the rule (which is actually the case in some settings hence the classification as chaotic). We cannot, obviously, change the past. We are where we are now. Unfortunately, or fortunately, we cannot undo many things in our lives, those things that heavily influenced the nature of the cross we have to bear at this point. I know, first-hand. It is unfortunate, but there's nothing much we can do about what has already transpired. It may be obvious to some, but it needs reiteration for a few others who need to deal with the healthcare-inflicted wounds of the past. Even if our protests and strikes do not deliver the results we are made to believe we are entitled to receive, our continual breakdown of service delivery infrastructure and operational devices is not going to make things better. In fact, it keeps on getting worse. Only a small number of countries are able to provide the majority of their citizens with the type of services and products that would warrant none of these resistive public uprisings.

How will the situation get better if patients keep on demanding *more* than what the government and public service sectors can provide? How will healthcare service improve if doctors are continually striking because they want better wages – they already get paid more than most others in the occupational world? Where will the money for increased wages come from? How will our healthcare systems improve if doctors are allowed to move whenever they become fed-up of working for "very small salaries" and under "conditions with very little incentives for retention"? Indeed, we do have a global catastrophe on our hands, but luckily it's not like a nuclear bomb that can actually kill people in an instant. It will kill people over a longer time, in terms of smashing the hopes for a better life, and actually decreasing the effectiveness of modern medicine to the point that more people will die earlier due to an elevation in the severity of their chronic conditions. Some will not think this to be the case, and instead will focus on the increases in longevity in richer societies. But extrapolation of current trends in chronic drug use and medications show a different picture. We already know how depressed the general populace has come to be, can we imagine how much worse it will get if we continue with the same behaviors we've been displaying for the last twenty or thirty years?

So, to return to figuring out where we stand, this is it: we have a chaotic state of affairs in most of our westernized healthcare settings. Most doctors, nurses, cleaners, staff members, patients, visitors and other guests are not too happy about the healthcare facilities or services, or both. If we're not complaining about service, we complain about money. If money's not the issue we complain about the attitude and nonchalant behavior of those who provide us the services. Strangely, we don't complain about our own similar behaviors, or other types of seemingly protective mannerisms, for example ignorance and blatant denial. If the attitudes of those healthcare personnel are not too problematic we tend to complain about government policies and other healthcare-related issues that impact of the softer side of society – the racism, ethnic preferences, status differentials and those kinds of stuff. Most of us are not even aware of nurses, doctors and other professionals who are severely compromised in their abilities to cope with patient loads, continual professional development and other factors that are not visible to those 'on the outside'. There are many who ultimately leave the healthcare workforce due to the status-based discrimination that occurs with every waking moment of a healthcare setting's operational effort, to assume jobs in other sectors of the occupational domain that don't perhaps need them as much as the sector they care to abandon. Perhaps the description seem dramatized, but rest assured that in many cases it would fall short by light years in capturing the real intensity of interpersonal dramas and conflict that characterize our hospital and clinic environments – this much is certain in quite a number of facilities in developed nations and almost all facilities in developing nations (of course, developing nations are hit harder because they tend to lose more human resources due to, for example, weakened competitiveness in terms of salaries and benefits).

By immersing oneself in the healthcare setting on a daily basis, continually over a number of weeks or months, the patterns emerge and the real motives behind certain behaviors become apparent; patience run out as more patients run in, sometimes the same gnawing patients, sometimes the same resource-based weaknesses of the system revealed – it affects those who are expected to offer the service with a smile, it affects those who need better and more efficient service but who cannot get it. It's almost like a jungle experience where the law of survival-of-the-fittest, a long-standing principle in nature, will apply in all of its brutality. This is how most healthcare situations are, at least from a public health perspective, in terms of what public facilities can offer. (For some, I suppose, it is perhaps better on the private side of medical service delivery and products). In the end, somewhere, somehow, a crack will appear. In some cases, already, the cracks are too wide. And as all the cracks across the whole face of Planet Healthcare start to merge, we're surely moving towards a catastrophic meltdown.

So, what can we do? Well, firstly, it depends on our identity. Are we the agents or the system? If we're part of both, then we're trapped. Our approach, as a start, will depend on which side of the coin we stand: as agents that provide the service or product; or as the system, the larger body of the two sides, those whom receive the professional service. As agents, it has been shown in the past (cf. Talcott Parsons) that we are not in the position to help ourselves out of the mess we're in. We lost control and are currently those who perpetuate what has been done before, we do as we were trained to do, most not knowing that a great mind of capitalistic dominance has indeed enshrouded us all into believing what we were taught to believe. Thus, the agents cannot help themselves (as they themselves have shown), they therefore need help, and for this the world's authorities have to step in: the medical qualifications framework must be adapted to suit a changing new world, and title-based supremacy within public healthcare settings must come to a grinding halt. The more important aspect within this reshaping is an equalization of status across the entire occupational landscape, so that the same amount and intensity of training across ANY discipline in life yield similar status-based titles, added to the idea that no person can be called a "Doctor" without publishing a doctoral dissertation or a series of peer-reviewed articles that signify a major contribution to the respective field of expertise. This, as a result, would be the first step, on behalf of the agents – it must be done by those who control how agents become agents – we cannot expect the agents to help themselves. They have proven inadequate, instead, by helping themselves to wealth and undeserved levels of status at the expense of the efforts of others. It would not be most appropriate, for the purposes of this volume, to suggest any practical steps on exactly how this reshaping of medical qualifications frameworks will be done – for that purpose, the world's authorities need to engage in meaningful discussions to advise on how to proceed. As a matter of urgency, it should be done sooner than later.

We should rather focus on the system, those of us who form the general populations in need of decent and affordable healthcare services and products. As consumers of healthcare services and products we reserve the right to be treated with equal respect, as fellow human beings deserving of the greatest amount of accountability. After all, it is our healthcare needs that give rise to the existence of the system. Yes, we form the system. This means that we have a sense of power, a measure of force. Because we form the system, we can also un-form it! Yes, we can undo the formation of the system – if we really, really, really want to do so. This is a mathematical logic of life – if you created something, then you can destroy it. Many other book writers have tried their best to convey the power we have within ourselves to create the kind of life for ourselves that we always dreamt about. "Power of the mind" is what most call it; some say "The Secret" or the "Law of Attraction". For most regular readers these terms will be familiar. Let's use them in assessment of our healthcare situation: we created a system of orthodox medicine to serve our needs of healthcare; when the system of healthcare does not provide what we need most (i.e. proper healthcare), we need to exert the necessary pressure to obtain from it what we need else we must destroy it. It follows that we find ourselves in this situation where the agent is not providing what the system needs; are we left with any other choice but to destroy the system, if the current system is beyond rescue?

How do we destroy our very own creation? This sounds pretty absurd. Well, if we accept that our healthcare needs are the reasons for establishing the current mode of healthcare systems around the world (from a western, orthodox point of view), then we can surely destroy that system by changing our healthcare needs. You don't have to destroy yourself, literally – you just have to change your needs. And this change of needs would be the first major realization in our effort to affect the rest of our lives with a greater sense of health. As global citizens, we can change the entire health landscape by changing the level and intensity of our need for orthodox medicine. The first major realization will help to unshackle us from the tiresome load we've been carrying for so many years. This realization must happen before we'll be empowered enough to take the first steps into a better state of healthcare for all. At this point we can start to appreciate any sentiment that relates the success of the greatest medical empire on our dependencies. We are so dependent hence the great success of the vast network of medical services and products – it is a simple supply-demand situation. The more dependent we became, the more supply provisions were made, and once we were so reliant on the provision, it gradually became more expensive with us not even noticing our addiction to the pharmaceutical release of the next new, more 'effective' drug.

We are collectively responsible for creating the system that is no longer serving in our best interests unless we profit from it, economically. Yes, some of us are economically healthier, but we are not healthy at all. We have such severe increases in prevalence of obesity, trauma, chronic conditions and terminal illnesses; it surely does deserve the labeling of catastrophic. How can we ignore it? How can we be happy about it? My parents cannot live one single day without medicine from the pharmacy; I am informed enough to guide them to a much better state of living, but they believe in the power of the generic prescriptions – already having lost its effects two decades ago. A sixty-year old grown-up cannot listen to advice about eating habits that will drastically reduce the need for those medications; it is sad to witness. How many people do you know around you with diabetes? Cancer? Heart and circulatory problems? The list is endless, not even to mention fetal alcohol syndrome, metabolic syndrome and drug-induced conditions. As mentioned before, it is very, very late for some of us to make the appropriate changes to cancel our conditions; for some it would be impossible.

If we lived all our lives in a reactionary mode, it will be very difficult to understand the idea of incorporating proactive measures and means of living to counteract the existence of disease and sickness in our lives. But whether or not it's too late for us in our very own situations, we should own up and make an effort to install a different sense of living into those around us, especially those born from us. When saying our needs can change the system, the idea that I wish to convey is simply that we can teach ourselves to become much less dependent on our doctors for advice, counsel and medication. If we need them now (as we've done in the past) it most probably is because we've been raised to believe that we need to go to the doctor with anything and everything medically related, and that no one knows better than the doctor. Now, we need to change this view, and we need to open ourselves up to the idea that orthodox doctors are no longer the most knowledgeable on issues of healthcare. They are knowledgeable with regards to most general aspects of western medicine, but they know very little about other conceptualizations of healthcare that otherwisely could have benefitted your life in the most amazing sort of ways. Sometimes, even – it's sad to admit – your western doctor knows much less about your condition than you could ever imagine. You need to do half a day's worth of proper web-based research, and you'll probably come to the same conclusion as him or her, for the majority of cases. This is no misnomer on my part. I have tested this for more than twenty years, and only in two cases did a doctor prove to me that my internet-based acquisition of knowledge could not beat experience. (Before internet was around, I had my mother to ask before we would consult the doctor, she was a nurse, and therefore my 'internet'). We are living in the information age; information is readily available. This is not just a slogan. Buy yourself a decent smartphone, and you'll be amazed at the power of having medical information downloaded in a second. I'm sure that one of these days you'll have a mass market of online doctors who'll dispense information with the same or better efficiency than those doctors for whom you have to sit in a queue for (there are already online medical services, but it's not yet mass market!).

Consumerism has really kept us bogged down, and had us rendered blind to the real, core issues within our busy lives. We must change our needs – simply because times have changed! Again. It keeps on changing. Only change is constant, remember? Yes, the system has expressed itself in almost every other facet of our lives – we need doctor's prescriptions to show at work when we're very lazy or overworked, or we need the syrup-based cold medicine just to make us feel better (it's like when we got to taste the sweet medicine when we were kids).

How do we change our needs? How do we become more independent? Since this is the information age we're living in, we need to get some information. Start by reading up on the medical industry, and all the political battles between different modes of medicine, and about orthodox medicine's lousy claim to superior authority. Yes, they are the only medicine professionals with legal backing in most court cases around the world, but they're also slowly losing to a more progressive advancement of holistic healing, CAM (complementary and alternative medicine) and integrative medicine. Germany is probably the one orthodox country showing the greatest support for CAM; it would be worth a sizeable bout of research. The fact that 'doctors' in the non-orthodox paradigms do not have as much state-accredited backing does not mean they don't know medicine. In some cases, they actually understand your ailments to the degree where they can offer immediate cures, instead of ones that hope to work, where instead orthodox practitioners mostly pray that your body don't reject it.

The one area of orthodox medicine, that makes it stand out from the pack of modes of medicine, is surgery. Yes, for sure, you need to be very highly trained if you're going to cutting into people for some of those operations that go far beyond the territory of routine surgeries; but for this reason surgery can be separated from the remainder of orthodox medicine's disciplines. It is a very telling aspect of the other approaches to medicine that they don't focus that much on surgical techniques and operations as a means of healing. The very ethos, then, is based on the idea that healthcare is a more holistic enterprise, and it follows that if your life is lived in accordance with understanding more of the environment's impact on your body, you could look forward to having a decreased need for surgery – because your body was treated differently and you showed more responsibility toward your health. This is ultimately where we're heading. The information age makes this possible. Before the 1990s it was difficult to find information about any field outside your domain of expertise; now the internet and the various folds of increased access to information have changed our lives. Hopefully, for the better. Sadly, for doctors and some other professionals who still feel they know it all, this is not good news. If your clients enter your consultation room with more information than you, then you do not deserve to be called doctor. Countries like China know why they heavily control access to information; information makes people powerful. Most governments know this and would usually want to prevent people from empowering themselves. Reading this book, for example, will get many people to rethink their health strategies. If it was twenty years ago, I would never be allowed to publish this book and most of what I had to say would fall on deaf ears of experts who's titles and labels will have prevented them from learning about things outside their comfort zones.

Your responsibility is to find the information that can inform on your own, personal situation, and that can help you making better decisions for your life. On the other hand, with more knowledge comes greater responsibility. Although you would be more informed about your health, you should also know that your abilities are also limited. You cannot claim to be an expert unless you are properly qualified to do so, after rigorous training and appropriate certification. The terms "expert advice" and "quality consultants" have sadly become subjected to literary prostitution, where virtually every new website proclaims some kinds of expertise without any real, tangible proof of authority. Yes, it's the information age, and knowledge is more readily available, but we must learn to use only what is of best application within our lives. How do we achieve this? We read, do research, write our questions, and formulate best practice models for our lives and those entrusted under our care. After we do all this, we make appointments with the experts and verify the usefulness of our models. But we don't just visit one expert. We are consumers, remember? As a habit of lifestyle, we check and recheck, visiting at least three different professionals or professional institutions over time, as a means of arriving at the point where we can confidently assert that we have modes of operation in our lives that can stand the test of our environment's influence on us.

It is not just a one-time affair. It's a lifestyle habit, to be done every year, as a matter of fact, not only when we are sick. Such kind of behavior would constitute a healthy mindset, and when you indeed end up having medical situations, you'll be less prone to panic attacks and very impulsive decisions that can derail any good effort that you may have made up to the point of being challenged. And we certainly have the right to question the credentials of those we seek advice from. Ask the medical professional to show any medical publications they published themselves, or any related scientific area of research they made a contribution to. This will allow you to have more confidence in them, for only in research enterprise does any individual really learn the art of understanding the basics of what they were trained to do. As a habitual response, develop a set of routine questions about your medication or medical situation – e.g. "what did I do to have this condition or what could I have done?", "where in the body does the medication act?", "what cells or organs are affected most?", "what are the known side effects of this medicine?", "what are the effects of other substance (e.g. coffee, tea, alcohol, smoking) while taking the prescribed medication", "what is the exact level of efficiency of this medication?", "is this the best medicine for my condition, and if not, why don't I receive the best medication if not for affordability?" – and so forth.

The idea here is shared not with the intention of never again using the services of medical professionals. We are people living in a more globalized society; it is as the movie made clear – contagion is always around us. We will always be prone to attacks on our immune systems and we'll not always be strong enough to ward off diseases that always surround us. We will always need those vital services and products for the sake of safeguarding our homes and families. This is the one positive result of the medicalizing of society – health is of central importance and we should make it one of the biggest priorities in our lives. This cannot be disputed, and should not be trifled with in any light-hearted manner. The intention of the preceding paragraphs is mainly to focus the individual's acceptance of his or her own status and importance in terms of providing medical care to self, first and foremost. Again, if it sounds too obvious to mention, then please take a look around in your present environment. How many people, to you knowledge, are taking care of themselves in very visible proportions? The experience in hospitals and clinics tell another story: if most of the people we know today had taken better care of themselves our limited means of healthcare infrastructure and resources would not be so strained and riddled with intense and complex politically-based policies and strictly state-approved scrutinized lists of protocols. It is very disheartening to see so many people walk around each day, some idle and some very productive, but indeed only a handful looking notably vibrant and energetic. In fact, the most alive and healthiest of people always seem to be the talking point in conversations. Their vibrance is disturbing to some others who happen to cross their paths at any given moment in life. A possible conclusion from this is that it has become the norm to be slouchy and borderline presentable, hiding the diseased expressions behind layers of clothing and fashionable glasses; as opposed to the exception where people are healthy, vibrant and utterly full of oozing life force. The world has become estranged to situations where people (or children) play, have regular physical contact or just plainly look happy. This transformation of our society has been depicted in many movies and other forms of entertainment, and it somehow pleases the general populace to see an actor portray the state of mind they find themselves under on a daily basis.

All over the world, people talk about the *good old days*, which is a bit strange to hear. What was so different in those days? Was it perhaps the fact that people actually still took much better care of themselves, being less addictive to substances (alcohol and drugs)? It certainly begs a moderate degree of serious contemplation. If we were all so healthy, as we mostly say we are, does it make sense to have this overwhelming glooming picture of modern society? I think not. And on this matter I would disagree to the far ends of the world: something is very different about the way in which people are taking care of themselves – they've either started caring in much less obvious ways, or they've stopped caring; I would not be able to understand any single reasoning that is showing me how healthy and happy people are. I've been watching closely for the last twenty years, and I am certain that I've seen a very big change in people's behavior around me, as well as in appearances. My family is my best example and if I were to share the gory details of those transformations, you would be equally shocked. In the end, we have a responsibility toward ourselves and we cannot overlook it, even if it is difficult to talk about. We cannot neglect ourselves any farther into the future; it is time that we pick it all up and do our best to be accountable to ourselves and those in our family environments.

***

The doctors and nurses will always be there – medicine, to many, will remain a noble profession – but it cannot continue to dump ineffective service and a sub-quality of products through the current healthcare system, especially if patients are not able to pay the required fees. At this point it is not known whether the medical professional will heed to this public call of changing the healthcare qualifications frameworks for the sake of better service delivery, after all, only a critical mass of people and institutions around the world will be able to amass such a will to change. I am aware of the fact that not one single person will be able to do this, but this book is considered a start, a very necessary start! During 2012 the WFME (World Federation for Medical Education) planned to host a conference to discuss the PhD requirements for doctors, but it was suddenly canceled. It has been under discussion for a few years already, and the idea stemmed from research that showed that most medical doctors were not able to understand the research processes involved in medical research, especially when leadership was needed toward meeting the goals of many medical research projects. Publishing this book at this time (early 2014) is not accidental; for many years I had to patiently wait for the right kind of conversation at medical conferences before letting this idea out. Medical doctors will not listen to the advice of someone they don't consider better or more highly qualified. For this reason I share the information through this publication, intending to gather support for what I believe is the one main reason for me being a medical researcher. The world of internet-based publication opened up new avenues of sharing, and it is my intention to use it to the best of my ability, to spread the message of the biggest change in medical science since the dawn of modern technology.

In essence, I support the growth of the medical profession, after all, it provides the environment where I work best, but unfortunately the current state of affairs cannot be allowed to grow any further else it demolishes our health or what's left of it. As mentioned earlier, the medical professionals will always be there, but in order to provide a more comprehensive service, the occupational boundaries must certainly be relaxed in favor of more integrative service delivery and cooperation between different healthcare professionals across the healthcare domain. As constituents within the system, and as those who collectively form the system to which the healthcare agents are providing their services and products, we need to become more aware of our responsibility towards ourselves, and we should definitely own up to it. In no way am I saying this is going to be easy, but based on current evidence that is slowly becoming plentiful, it is possible for normal citizens to change the approach to health.

Once we accept this notion, namely that we are indeed most responsible for everything concerned with our health, then we are ready to take the first step: determine, using all resources at your current disposal, if you're using the most appropriate holistic approach to health. If you think your doctor knows more about your health than what you know yourself, then this is the first big situation that needs overturning. Find out about your condition, read about it, make appointments with professionals other than your doctor, and when you see your doctor, make sure to determine that you are doing everything possible to aid in best recovery, or that you're not being held down from recovery either due to a lack of knowledge or money. This type of investigation will possibly not give you all the answers you would hope for, but it will illustrate where you (and your immediate family) really stand in terms of your health. There are a number of people who already subscribe to this type of healthcare protocol, and their experiences, I bet, will corroborate the sense of *you* becoming *your* own best, most trusted healthcare professional.

In Volume 1 the issue of second opinions was discussed in detail, and it applies very directly to the situation referred to in this section. If this will be the first time in your life that you ventured toward seeking answers from doctors or knowledgeable professionals outside the normal confines of orthodox medicine, do not be fearful of what you may find. In fact, I would bet some hard-earned cash that some patients will find much less expensive and possible more effective solutions to healthcare problems they've had to endure for many years. This will help to add credence to the hypothesis that not all of the best solutions to health are found in orthodox medicine, and some solutions that are complex by orthodox reasoning may indeed be simpler to treat by other approaches, and could also cost significantly less. Note that I am not speaking out against orthodox medicine as a philosophy of medicine, but that I, categorically, speak against the claims by many western doctors that they have the best solutions for health, or that orthodox medicine is the best or should be the only legitimate approach to health. The progressive, modern world has moved a long way since those times during which herbalists were burned or prosecuted for being caught while allegedly practicing witchcraft. A pair of scented candles and moxibustion herbs still serve as the ultimate relaxer – it is by no means of witch-crafting that the candle's scent actually relaxes the nerves and muscles – but the mainstream medical fraternity will continue to denounce its very popular relaxation effects, because "it does not prove to cure disease", and also, I think, because it is something not invented by pioneers of western medicine, else it would have been part of its daily practices. In essence, at the base of all tension in the world of healthcare we still have fraternal mindsets at work that prevent us from achieving better health. But to the general Joe or Jill out there, do go ahead and try it for yourself. It will transform your idea of relaxation and could possible help to lower your blood pressure in ways that orthodox medicine cannot explain.

Once you know whether or not you've been receiving the most appropriate healthcare treatments and services, you will have taken Step 1, the step that starts your journey toward better health for you and those entrusted in your care.

The responsibility of your own health – and all matters related to it – is indeed a huge responsibility. To place it in context, imagine following all the medical information of your life since the moment you were born until you die; the charts, the emergencies, traumas and accidents. It's like being aware of yourself in so much more detail. It can be mind-boggling, but luckily we don't have to remember ALL of that. There are ways of making the remembering part a bit easier. First of all, you cannot monitor all of your health when born, or course, which means that someone else will do this for you. It will be your mom, dad, grandma, grandpa, an aunt, uncle, nanny, or some other person under whose care you've been placed, till you reach a certain age. This "certain age" will differ for different people, and brings up the complex issue of when anyone is really ready to undertake this sort of responsibility. For legal reasons this age of responsibility will vary between countries and cultures, but of more importance is to consider exactly when a growing individual begins to understand the idea of being aware and responsible for maintaining a state of health.

To my best knowledge, toddlers are already receptive to advice of this nature and they're already able to participate in issues of health – preventing wounds or taking care not to hurt themselves unnecessarily, taking care of wounds when they occur (even if just performing the act of notifying an adult in close range or calling an emergency number), not ingesting anything that could be dangerous to their young bodies, eating healthy foods and preventing the over-assumption of junk food or foodstuffs not considered healthy, knowing the basic parts of their anatomy by which they would be able to describe pain, being aware of the duty to report pain or any uncomfortable sensations in their bodily systems, being very aware of pain and how to convey any feelings of it, understanding that it's important for the adults to know when pain is experienced, and so forth. This stage, of being a toddler, would then represent the start of this health-conscious journey. Our homes and public institutions are currently swamped with toddlers and young children who live silent lives, for fear of shame, humiliation and other damning emotional embarrassments; if the future is going to be progressively different, this, obviously, would be the place to start. Most parents, admittedly, will not share their healthcare afflictions with their children, for obvious reasons, but imagine if your child grows up to be the kind of parent who shares with their kids matters of healthcare in a fact-of-matter way without having to feel ashamed, humiliated or embarrassed. That would be nothing short of a remarkable achievement if achieved on the scale of entire societies and, to judge by today's standards, would be something worth striving for. For most of our lives, we've been silent about some things that need not be dealt with in silence. Imagine the massive change in society when this silence is broken. If you teach your child to be responsible for his or her own health, and you show them exactly how it's done, your child will grow up knowing how to take care of themselves with a much greater level of effectiveness than before – our previous generations are not very capable of this level of sharing. If my parents were to fall ill today, I would only know a few days or weeks later; they fear being perceived as weak or frail, or any one of those other debilitating stigmatizations that generally prevent people from seeking help when its most needed, even while there's still time to influence the outcome where a clean bill of health is being threatened. What makes us weakest is what we think others perceive us to be. On the other hand, if you know you're a responsible individual that sometimes can fall sick, you will have no fear in seeking the speediest way to recovery even it means asking for help from other people. There is no shame in being interdependent. Humans were not made to be alone. For some reason, though, modern society has evolved to the state of preferring the solitude and silence, which perhaps is a more underlying reason for some of us failing to achieve more progressive states of health. No matter the technological progress we make, some things of being human will never change. We should never aspire to become like the robots we are proud to manufacture for we are social beings that need others for our overall well-being.

It is our responsibility to maintain our health and to thereby acknowledge our humanness, to live up to our need of healthcare for our happiness, and to understand the urgency by which we need to approach this matter. Strangely enough, at the beginning of the preceding paragraph the following were mentioned: "charts, emergencies, traumas and accidents". Is this really how we form a conceptualization of medical care? Do we remember the healthy times, when we did not see a doctor's office or consultation room as a result of some pressing medical need? This should make us think. Can you imagine the type of lifestyle not driven by a panic, a fear of some hypochondriac notion of dying because something is wrong with us? We are indeed crippled by a fear, a collective fear that has driven our world to where it is today – high levels of disease, war, crime. Even nature is upset, to judge by all the floods, earthquakes and other disasters. Our collective energies produced a rather sickly environment, and it is mainly to this sickliness that I am reacting. It makes me sick when I consider this position. Could it be that we've become so fearful that it reached a critical mass that swept over the world, even affecting nature? How could we allow it? Well, the answers are many, the purpose here is not to analyze all of these answers – the point is actually to establish whether we've been asking these questions and whether or not we're going to do anything to change things for the better, for our own sakes, first, and then for the sake of a more humane humanity.

***

Your medical doctor, technically, is not a healthcare provider; he or she is a professional that specializes in assisting people with achieving certain predefined outcomes for health; hopefully these outcomes are associated with a better quality of life (in terms of health) or plainly the removal of whatever obstacle to health may present itself in any recognizable form. Medical doctors, from a very technical point of view, don't care. The nursing profession was the heart of the caring industry. The doctor was always the nurse's superior; in those bygone days this arrangement was acceptable, but nowadays it impacts on the effectiveness of healthcare. Today, generally, people don't care about other people. If you think this is not true, then find one concrete example of genuine caring in your community that would show real, humane care without any tangible rewards attached to it. Not many such examples are found, and especially not in professional environments. You would see few such examples in homes of people, left with almost no resources, who suffer in silence. Many religious institutions exist that provide such community-based care. In fact, the policies of big organizations and businesses are written in such a way as to ensure the measurable extent

77

of free, care-based services, as a means of minimizing risk. It is not surprising, though. Consumers of services have really gone further than what was needed in terms of benefitting by those services, and many businesses would go bust if they were to be more *caring*.

The crux of this conjecture is mainly that we need a new term that describe what medical people are doing; medical care is no longer appropriate, expect for a very small percentage of cases. Even healthcare, as a term, seem insufficient. If you don't have enough financial backing, the people at the hospital frown and some want to push you down the stairs instead of into the surgical room; if you do not qualify for that medical aid you are less likely to receive competent levels of professional service. I am not convinced that caring is the most appropriate term for use in contemporary medicine; we must find another term. Medical assistance or health assistance could be better terms; the medical professional is the person to provide medical advice that could assist in alleviating the problem or assist by providing a reference to where better or more effective service could be found. There's no shame in not being able to provide the client with what's needed; there's much shame in pretending that you know exactly how to take care of matters. Even if it pains me to acknowledge it, many nurses, too, stopped caring. I've seen nurses and patients fight, especially when the doctors' are not around to supervise and take charge; it's incredible how the ethos in the caring industry came to change since the 1990s. The terms medical professional and caring professional can be used for those who specialized in medicine and nursing, respectively. In fact, the roles of each should be clarified more succinctly so that senior caring professionals can enjoy exactly the same status and rank as the senior medical professionals. This will indeed be a challenge to implement, but it stands to reason that such change will motivate more conscientious people to invest careers in the healthcare fraternity, as we would need for the next millennium. Equally, the other professionals in the healthcare domain can named according to their main function, e.g. internal medicine professional, rehabilitation professional, therapeutic professional, and so forth. The names are not as important as the realization that the term caring should be used with caution. I would mainly choose to focus on the words, titles and terms used within the hospital and clinic settings; those other, higher-level terms in politics and economics can be discussed elsewhere and at another point in time. The essential element here is extracting the notion that the caring industry is not living up to its preached ethos, and that *something's gotta go* – a more appropriate job title would be a great start.

***

"You should take care of yourself".

Now this statement should make more sense. And it should appeal to you on a different level than before. If you use the term healthcare, you are talking about yourself: me and you, not them, us or we. This is the important step: to realize that we are primarily responsible for our own healthcare, and when we cannot help ourselves to better states of health, we consult those trained to assist us in providing ourselves with care. I cannot rely on you to care for me. I can rely on you to help me take care of myself by sharing your expertise, if you are indeed trained to that level of professionalism. Here included here is a shift of awareness, a small shift perhaps, but a very meaningful one. Medical professionals will specialize in providing assistance in medical matters, nursing professionals will specialize in providing assistance in caring matters – medical interventions are separated from caring interventions although a very strong interrelationship is implied. In the same manner pharmaceutical professionals will specialize in matters of pharmaceutical nature; therapeutic professionals will provide therapeutic advice and interventions; and so forth. But it is you who will supervise your healthcare, and who will take charge of anything pertaining to your healthcare. You cannot leave it to people who don't care about you. Only if I have shown to care for you in your daily life and over a substantial period of time, and if we have a strong interpersonal relationship, then I would qualify, perhaps, to help you care for yourself, but even then I would never be able to completely take care of you – I have myself to completely care for. Healthcare is a personal matter, and the modern plague of consumerism cannot be allowed to take away from you even your health.

This is the step we all should take. Some have taken this step already, and over them medical institutions have no hold. As a globalizing society of individuals we are in a position to share the knowledge that will help us to take better care of ourselves; away from empty consumerism that cannot alleviate our most pressing healthcare needs. A sound state of health pervades and motivates every other aspect of your life, in the same that being sick also overrides everything else. It's a matter of choice, really, even if you cannot allow yourself to agree with that, for now. We all have choices to make, and to be healthy is a choice that you should make. You have a better chance of making this choice if your ancestors already paved the way. If, however, you are the first in your family tree, it cannot be easy to accept that you have a choice. We have, since the times of rife colonialism, accepted what has been handed down to us; and those colonialist minds are the same that would perpetuate the reliance on orthodox medical provision. Surely, the world is changing at a faster pace than ever before, and it is no ordinary chance that a book such as this would be in your hands, or on your electronic device, to be read conscientiously and for your benefit. Step up and make the better choice; become your own best provider of healthcare, and arm yourself up against those powers that seek to carefully maintain your disease-ridden state.

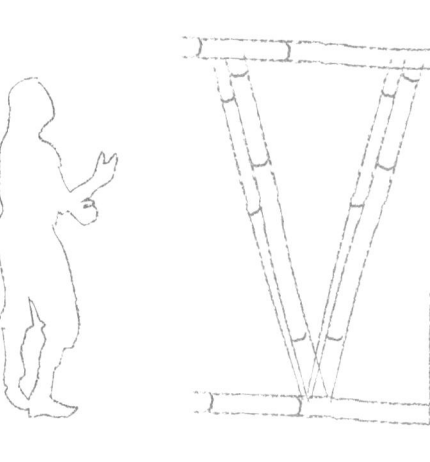

"From birth, man carries the weight of gravity on his shoulders.
He is bolted to earth.
But man has only to sink beneath the surface and he is free."

Jacques Yves Cousteau

seventh STONE

The chapter title implies something heavy, such as in the Old English reference in terms of measuring the mass of an object or someone's weight. A certain heaviness envelopes us, usually, when talking about matters this serious. For many years we've tried to unravel many complex issues in healthcare and, to many people, after reading this book, a different perspective will altogether emerge. This perspective may strengthen the path of progress towards better health for all, but in a different sense as the discussions of President Obama and other leaders in healthcare over the last few years. It is a heavy topic, if I may, but the heaviness must eventually dissipate as we collectively lift ourselves out of the deep pits of uncertainty and desperation about issues of how we're going to take better care of ourselves. If you are heavier, you have more inertia; it will be more difficult for you to move away from where you've been up to this point in time. After doing the dependence-exercise (see Table 2), we have to decide what to leave behind as we move ahead. Captain Simon says it's time to throw some things overboard; we need to make the ship lighter else we sink, and our legacy will be lost forever. Too many ships have been sinking to the deepest ridges along the ocean floor, but we cannot allow our vessels of healthcare to follow suit. Yes, we have to throw things that make us heavier, but we cannot throw it all – some things are needed for the tumultuous journey ahead. But how do we know which things to throw or not? Well, let's have a more pragmatic appraisal of our situation. All hands on deck.

One way of knowing what you don't need is to decide the things that you really, really need. Some people

Table 2 Dependence Exercise

Questions to gauge dependency on orthodox medicine's services and products	Answer (please encircle your choice)
1. Do you need to go to the hospital or clinic every week or month?	yes / maybe / no
2. Do you need to see the (western) doctor every week or month?	yes / maybe / no
3. If you don't see the doctor every week or month, will you still be able to function normally, e.g. going to work every day, doing exercises, performing chores?	yes / maybe / no
4. If you go for medical assistance, must you always see a doctor? (see question 5 below)	yes / maybe / no
5. If you go for medical assistance, are you adequately served by medical staff of lower rank than a doctor?	yes / maybe / no
6. Do you agree: "I cannot function optimally without my prescribed medicine"?	yes / maybe / no
7. Do you agree: "if my medicine is taken away I'll be very sick"?	yes / maybe / no
8. Do you agree: "there is no hope for better health if my family or I stop our weekly or monthly visits to the clinic"?	yes / maybe / no
9. Over the last five years have you seen the inside of medical facility less than twice per year?	yes / maybe / no
10. Over the last five years have you received medication for any purpose less than twice per year?	yes / maybe / no
11. Do you agree: "I can function optimally without much assistance from any healthcare providers"?	yes / maybe / no

Key to interpretation:
If you answer "yes" or "maybe" to five questions from questions 1 through 8, then you are *very dependent* on orthodox medical provision. If you answer "yes" or "maybe" to three or four questions from that range, then you are *mildly dependent* on orthodox medical provision. Answering "yes" to at least 2 of the 3 questions from questions 9 through 11 renders you *not dependent* on orthodox medical provisions. Answering "yes" to question 5 could mean that you may be more dependent on specific services offered exclusively by doctors as opposed to services offered by lower-ranked healthcare personnel, which adds to your dependency on orthodox medical provision.

will have 'needs assessment' pop into some part of the mind, but what we want to achieve is more than just a mere assessment: we have to assess our needs and also know how we're going to use what we plan to keep (if we have it) or how to get it (if we don't yet have it); all else must be discarded. If we cannot know how we'll use it, it will not be useful at all. In order to kick-start this journey – as with many things in today's wonderful world of the web – enter your search terms into a web-based search window. The two words making up today's theme are "health needs". After doing as instructed, using Yahoo! (on 1 November 2012), the first three links appeared: "*Health needs assessment: A practical guide*", "*Development and importance of health needs assessment*" (you have to scroll to the 8th page of the PDF-document to see the relevant article), and "*What Is a Health Needs Assessment? | eHow.com*". This already provides us with so much to start with; it also shows the serious level of work involved in making this kind of information more accessible to the public. In fact, this book is nothing more than a more personalized effort to do exactly the same – to get this kind of information to people that will benefit by having it. But wait, there is something more interesting – if you look toward the top of the page, just above the listed links, there's a section marked "*Also try...*", listing other links connected to your search, viz.

mental health needs	children with special health needs
health needs of the elderly	community health needs
health needs a hero	home health needs
health needs analysis	basic health needs
health needs survey	public health needs

You see, the concept of health needs is an all-encompassing concept, and this is something that could add much unnecessary weight to your stone if not properly dealt with. Literally, if you don't treat the matter of healthcare with the necessary levels of respect and interest, it will weigh you down – not only you, but those who live with you and those close enough to you to care about your welfare. No person is strong enough to carry it all, but every person can be equipped to make the more appropriate selection that will benefit them more directly, individually, especially in terms of maintaining a state of health by which a more pleasing life could be lived, given the other restraints that we all experience, to more or lesser extents. We all want a "good" or "exceptional" state of health; but for each of us it is different. A fully functional, disease-free state of health could thus be thought of as being a type of personality; we each have our own unique set of requirements, but with some basic similarities that could broadly be applied to any person (e.g. clean water, decent-quality food, adequate sleep and exercise, etc.). No single approach will be relevant to all, but all of us can benefit immensely by acute learning of what pertains to us individually, taken from the whole spectrum of what is available in our environments. Some others may even compare healthcare to religion, whereby a certain kind of health can be achieve by living according to certain set of rules that serve to achieve a predetermined set out of outcomes which may underscore the individual's philosophy and beliefs on life.

Whatever the approach, it must remain as conclusion that healthcare is an individualized notion whereby the individual decides for him or herself about how best to cope with such a huge responsibility and how best to deal with finding external assistance in the event that self-management of healthcare becomes challenged outside the comfort zones of the respective individual's usual frame of reference. Losing the ability to manage your own state of health predisposes you to offload the responsibility thereof onto professionals in the business of healthcare, most of whom have lost the humane approach, and most of whom are not adequately prepared to handle both your and their own individual loads. This is where the stone becomes too heavy (the individual load has been amplified), and at this point the Captain has no choice but to throw you into the sea together with the excess cargo created in the process of inadequate management of duty and responsibility.

Let's survey the global lands for some proofs of things currently in place, or not in place, that can help us relinquish some of the heavier weights. One of the striking developments in Europe comes in the form of the Alliance of Scientific Organizations, operated under the auspices of the German Federal Minister of Education and Research. This project, called *High-Tech Strategy 2020*, is massive in its scope and expected levels of expenditure over the next few years; it aims to position Germany as a global leader in terms of five major areas, namely (i) climate and energy, (ii) health and nutrition, (iii) mobility, (iv) security, and (v) communication. The group responsible for healthcare and health-related research published an online brochure (titled *Researching: Health*) that contains meaningful statements of intent, also expressing a few thoughts that echo well within our renewed or refreshed conceptualization of healthcare. To underscore sentiments raised previously, a few quotes from their marketing brochure are provided below.

"Our health system ought actually to have a different name: ill-health system. When it comes to disease control, traditional medicine far too often waits for a condition to develop – in many cases until it is barely treatable or no longer treatable at all. The only real way out of this ingrained situation involves a radical rethink of medical practice and research: away from therapy and toward prevention."

"This includes a change in the behavior patterns of the general public, who must view their health as a competence and should visit their doctor regularly when they are healthy..."

"One way or another, the focus of research and of the 'health executives' must shift more towards the patient."

"In conversations with patients, five key components can be identified: the opening, the discussion of the symptoms, the diagnosis, the treatment planning and the conclusion of the conversation. The beginning in particular sets the scene – it is an essential element in building a relationship."

As we move toward 2020, our conceptualization of healthcare must indeed keep up with realities surrounding us, realities that are very different from realities in previous decades. In a manner of speaking, we would have to shed the old skin, like a snake does every once in a while. Only by shedding of the old skin can we appreciate the beauty of the new – a new way of thinking is perhaps the best thing we can allow ourselves to adopt in this unsure world post-2008. Many projects have been called to life in the last four or five years, all heading towards 2020, with renewed vigor and intent – but do you really think any of our current realities will change significantly? Maybe not. If the change does not occur on a very personal level for each individual, then surely all these new appraisals and visions of a better future will fall to naught, like many things before. Only a change of thinking can lead to a genuine change of behavior. By acting differently, we truly show ourselves capable of change.

Another striking development is contained in UK Parliament's Health and Social Care Act 2012, the promulgation of which is currently still laden with loads of raging controversy. Calls were made to change how the NHS (UK's publicly funded National Health Service) was controlling the practice of medicine, and this act was the current Secretary of State for Health's answer to the very demanding issue, an issue that characterized tensions across the British medical scene for more than two decades. Andrew Lansley's Act, as it is more commonly known, received the Royal Assent on 27 March 2012, which is one very big step closer to becoming enforced official legislation. Lansley denies claims of privatization of the UK's NHS whereas professional medical experts concluded that there are "evidence that privatization is an inevitable consequence of many of the policies contained in the Health and Social Care Bill" (Clive Peedell, British Medical Journal). When introducing the white paper to MPs, Lansley shared three key principles: placing the patients at the center of the NHS; changing the emphasis of measurement to clinical outcomes; and empowering health professionals, in particular GPs. When analyzing the intent of the proposed act, one is inclined to readily agree with the first two key principles – it seems that the Secretary of State for Health did a fair bit of research about the current states of health around the world – but it seems ludicrous that GPs should be empowered even more than what is presently the case. At this point it's not exactly clear how GPs could be empowered even more (our prior analysis led us to conclude that GPs were already over-empowered), but a strong warning bell sounds at this realization: as globalized citizens we need to become more aware of what we can expect from the healthcare providers in our environments, whether they're state-funded or privatized. No matter how we look at it, the "empowerment" clause is almost certainly never attached to the "patient" term. Thus, the necessary reiteration: as individuals we need to change the way we look at our health; we need to change the way we take care of ourselves; we are our own best healthcare providers. If the UK government approves this act, it will surely allow healthcare policies to continually benefit the GPs more than what it is benefitting the patients (as is the current status quo), even if it provides some emotional comfort by stating as a key principle the intent to make patients the center of the NHS. If you make the patient the center, then you do not empower the GP. These are two mutually exclusive concepts.

If you make the patient the center of your healthcare system, then you must empower the patient first. For the individual in need of improved health, it remains best to empower yourself first and foremost; by taking the responsibility of your own health upon yourself, you need not subject yourself to the political will of those who continually seek to harvest a capitalistic profit from the healthcare system to which they are supposed to render a public service. Allowing the state to continually empower GPs could be our own contribution to increasing the weight on our stones. This issue alone raises many more within the holistic debate regarding status of medical doctors, but it suffices to say here that very strong resistance to politicians is needed if there are any real hopes of changing our healthcare systems into systems that really cater for its people instead of its professionals. By empowering ourselves – individually, holistically, inwardly, and spiritually – we can indeed offer the necessary anti-force to the agent that does not serve in the best interest of the system upon which it is acting, and from which it is greatly benefitting.

In a more liberal appraisal of the state of healthcare, if compared to Lansley, Felix Unger (currently the President: European Academy of Science and Arts) published an article (*Health is Wealth: Considerations to European Healthcare, 2012*), asserting that "Healthcare provision is developing from a National to a European endeavour as a European Healthcare Market (EHCM) serving its people, legitimized by the European Convention, which sets out the principals of a socio-market economy, competition and self-responsibility". Further, he states:

"In many countries Healthcare is considered as a part of social welfare and has a very high political priority, which creates a national state-monopoly with a few private exceptions. This is a source of mismanagement and discomfort to patients. Europe is now ready to form a European market for Healthcare with the essential prerequisite "Health for All" as a part of our culture. This market depends on clinical leadership."

For our purposes, two concepts are highlighted from Unger's publication: *self-responsibility* and *Health for All*. The Europeans, for many decades now, have been world leaders in many respects, and in terms of sharing resources across borders this is particularly true. Within today's milieu of multiculturalism, there is simply no better philosophy to guide our steps into the future: we need to relax our idea of nationalism for the sake of improved health. You immediate environment is going to become more multicultural – this is the way the world is moving – and to accommodate issues of health, you need to relax your personal restrictions on what you share in public and how you share it. Governments have a dual responsibility – toward their own people and to those from the outside who wish to live within those particular borders. Unger states that considerations of nationalism are placed second to considerations of continental or regional associations, which indicates a progressive step toward globalization from a governmental point of view. It usually takes a bit longer for masses of people to align to the governmental approaches (if accepted on the part of the masses) but it is nonetheless a step in the better direction.

The term *Health for ALL* now become a poignant point of interest, or a welcoming phrase of the future – it just depends on which side of the line you decide to stand. Of course, this book advocates for the welcoming aspect within that phrases, in that we are all becoming more responsible for our own health; while doing so we are more open to sharing the resources that our governments have placed at our disposal. Our governments can control how many people enter our borders whereas we control how dependent we are on those resources and how willing we are to share with outsiders. A healthy interplay can exist to benefit more people in more settings. It is not impossible. This term *'Health for All'*, or *'Healthcare for ALL'*, thus encapsulates many different layers of acceptance and realizations about health and healthcare, and becomes a guiding light as we enter a new dispensation of healthcare. Furthermore, Unger does not shy away from admitting that privatization is inevitable, given the many huge pressure differentials that load governments with tasks and responsibility they forever struggle to fulfill. In fact, he cites Chassard and Quintin, who already in 1992 predicted the growing importance of privatization within healthcare and that future co-payment options will be unavoidable! Unger's model is divided into three clusters: medical arts, medical organizations and financing. He uses a triangle to pictorially illustrate the concept with the patient at the heart of the triangle, in similar conceptual fashion as Lansley in the latter's offering of a key principle placing the patient at the heart of the NHS. Ultimately, Unger's conclusion is concise and aptly stated: "At the beginning of the 21st century the patient has become more independent and self-motivated. The trend is towards the provision of medical services based on the patients' own responsibility in a free market".

In a free market we have more power in deciding how we load or offload our stones. Yet carry we must. If the governments want to make it easier to carry, then let's welcome it by all means; let's not accept the conditions where it's made easier for us to be dependent on the assistance on offer. If the government is for the people, let it be for the independence of its people while providing what it can and making sure that the basic services come at the most reasonable premium; if it thrives on deep, perpetual dependence of its people, it should not be a government at all or it should not claim to place its people at the center of revised conceptualizations that live up to be no more than renewed attempts of nonsense political lip service.

Unger also states that "this market depends on clinical leadership." To this specific point we might take exception. If we consider that medicine (as a profession) is no longer to be pre-eminent amongst the healthcare professions, then we can also consider the idea that healthcare leadership is not solely based on what the clinical domain of medicine has in its plan for the future of healthcare. It is constructions such as these that perpetually prevent many politicians and healthcare leadership from understanding how medical dominance was able to have its hold on the healthcare world. We can no longer stay ignorant of these matters.

In America, there's Obama and his healthcare act which has gripped the best of imaginations across the globe since his first year (2008) as US president. What is so captivating about Obama and his presidential campaign, and what has really transpired the last five years (the first of Obama's two terms) to have culminated in the "most retweeted tweet ever"? (Obama's 2012 victory tweet broke all previous records on the Twitter website). Let me attempt an answer: the USA has the most expensive medical service in the world – it outranks everyone else, even China – and this despite being a developed country. Leonard J. Weber, a medical ethicist, said in 2001 that "good-quality healthcare means cost-effective healthcare", but "more expensive healthcare does not mean higher-quality healthcare" and "certain minimum standards of quality must be met for all patients" regardless of health insurance status. In effect, Obama is promising to achieve something that up till now was not achievable on American soil for a long number of years – to stop America from being the most expensive in terms of healthcare and to assist the poorest of people to a decent level of medical care. These are stupendously huge claims to make and cannot, in my opinion, happen in two terms of presidential office. Firstly, Obama will have to consider the idea of remaining in charge of health for a long number of years after his presidency to achieve what he is claiming to be able to achieve during his presidency. Secondly, the world has always looked to Europe and America for global leadership, but since China's rise to the top of the world in terms of GDP-based economic strength, things have changed: Europe (as a whole) is not impressed by Obama's victory; Asia (through ASEAN) is looking to build stronger ties with an Obama-based administration, especially after work done by Hilary Clinton; and some of the other lesser but economically significant countries are looking to some parts of Europe and Australia for leadership, instead of America. Thirdly, the Obama Administration is made up of experts who mostly received their training during the hey-day years, and who cannot show the leadership needed for integration on the world stage especially considering the demand for expertise in dealing with people from the East. The former glory days of America were based on, or depended on, peoples' perceived economic superiority of the USA; however, in the knowledge-driven world new and better leaders are born elsewhere and can provide more effective solutions across a wider demographic than what the USA has been able to do more recently. In Obama's favor, the USA drives web-based technology and associated enterprises; the dollar is still the international preference as trading currency; the American culture revolution still has firm establishments in many humble places across the world; these are factors that will continue to drive America's domination in certain world events, but the half-life has been reached and the demise of this domination is in sight. Therefore, we need to look at the Obama more closely, in an attempt to understand how his philosophy, as a political proponent of more affordable healthcare, can help us toward *Healthcare for ALL*, or whether it will help us at all. In essence, can Obama and his approach help us carrying our stones? Let's investigate.

Heart disease is America's number-one killer. More Americans die from this wretched affliction than any other disease on American soil or in American air. Pay attention: this is America's biggest killer. When you consider the Obama-Biden Plan, you'll notice without any effort that it cannot really be called a healthcare plan; it is more befitting to call it a healthcare financing plan.

Healthcare involves more than financing. That's pretty obvious. Now, consider a 2012-publication that says *"Study Shows More Than Half of All Americans Will Get Heart Disease"*. Does the Obama-Biden Plan address the issue of heart disease and its prevention in any serious detail? Why not? Well, the Obama Campaign for presidency is a very good campaign – it showed itself spectacularly during the 2012 elections; and even in the victory speech Obama had to mention that politics is important. People cheered him, but still more than fifty percent of Americans will continue to die due to heart disease and associated disorders. The reason for this being important is simply that Obama used a very secure political stage to allow his fellow, beloved Americans to believe that healthcare will finally be as affordable to even poorer people. During his victory speech he had to mention to the case of the young girl with leukemia and how she already benefitted from the Obamacare assistance; this is remarkable considered that the Affordable Care Act (PPACA) was only signed in during 2010 and constitutionally defended earlier during 2012. After the 2008 recession it is plainly obvious that any reduction of costs or increased financial benefit would sit well with voters; hence the neatly poised Obamacare plan. What most Americans don't seem to realize is that there's a very serious problem amongst them that need more attention, and no matter how much money you make available for healthcare financing, you could not solve America's number problem through Obama or his Obamacare plans. If you believe anything to the contrary, you are in for the shock of a lifetime.

The other more obvious thing is that, in more cases, the onset of heart disease is related to diet, lifestyle or work habit. If America wants to stop having heart disease, the average person will have to live a different kind of life, eat different kinds of food and perform different kinds of exercises on a daily, habitual basis. Heart disease happens to be a very expensive thing to treat for; it's no wonder that America has the most expensive healthcare system (wasn't that a bit obvious)! The PPACA, in essence, has a great intention, but it is not taking the real matter of health to the place where it belongs: in the mind of the average person must develop the idea that health is an individual responsibility, and that individual changes in daily behaviors will ultimately cause real healthcare to develop more effectively. The main issue here is that even if healthcare becomes more affordable (by whatever monetary standards you measure) does it really allow you to live a healthier life? Will it make you healthier knowing you can afford to see more doctors or get more prescriptions? It seems like whole generations of seemingly educated people are missing this one simple idea. What was labeled "Obama's Blindness" before can now become a global blindness when it comes to matters of health. This kind of blindness really makes the stone heavier; after the 2012 election it seems feasible to predict that this stone is going to become heavier than the planet itself before we really allow ourselves to see the other side more clearly. We are resistant to change and perhaps our resistance is the leading cause of disease and poor states of health. The Obamacare assistance cannot make this stone lighter: at best, it will motivate you to carry the stone for longer; at worst, you will not see that day coming when the heavier stone will pull you down into a pit from which you can never free yourself.

Down south, the Australian Government's Preventative Health Taskforce released a document titled *Australia: The Healthiest Country by 2020*. This is no small challenge to mount, but if you consider that Australia has recently been voted to be "the best country to live in" then it may be a worthy conjecture when stating that the Australians have the best chance of achieving this feat, to judge by the definitions and scope of operations as contained in the very detailed document (freely available online). Indeed, Australia has been known for showing the way forward in many respects; taking into consideration their current stance on developing better resources and infrastructure in rural and remote areas across the vast Australian landscapes, they may well already be one of the healthiest nations, at least in terms of their openness to learning about health and the necessary requirements for staying healthy. On page 44 in the online statement of action, a paragraph is headed with the admonishment "*Act early throughout life*", a statement that serves to underscore the main thrust of holistic preventative medicine. This has been said many times before – we know the saying "prevention is better than cure" – but in itself the statement did not represent a guiding philosophy for many nations in terms of public health provision. Until now, that is. Curative medicine fought a raging battle for survival, but it is ultimately the preventative philosophies that must prevail. Curative mindsets have become too capitalistic whereas the preventative mindsets will help citizens across the world to develop lifestyles without forced, helpless dependence on governmental or privatized, profit-seeking enterprises. Further contextualization occurs through the following statements:

"Early childhood experiences may place children on health and developmental pathways that are costly and difficult to change. Therefore, children necessarily form the cornerstone of any prevention agenda."

This is not new knowledge – countries such as Cuba have already paved the way for successful establishment of primary care-based, preventative healthcare systems. It is just a matter of political will that prevents many other nations to follow suit. If one understands that political will is attached to economic profitability and issues of access to wealthier lifestyles for a select few, then one can easily comprehend how difficult the required changes will be for those who have benefitted most by previous healthcare agendas – those who would want to keep things as they are so that the benefits can accrue in better margins than before, if possible; or if change is inevitable, those who would agree to as little change as is needed for the profitability to remain close enough to justify their efforts within the healthcare environment. This is a simplified argument – it must be remembered that Cuba's success is attributed to The Revolution that started in 1959 – but we must not lose sight of the idea that such healthcare systems are possible. The Australians, as a nation of progressive-minded individuals, have shown that concerted alignment of will and effort can indeed produce changes on a massive scale that is large enough to benefit whole communities of people, even in areas with lower populations and wider geographical spread. If one considers children to be the cornerstone of prevention strategies for better health it follows that education systems also need the necessary overhaul that aligns it with the appropriate healthcare outcomes. Obama even committed to a reform of education in America (a tactic in his election campaign, perhaps), but instead has been inundated with the healthcare situation and must still show seriousness with regards to education. In this regard, Australia has moved ahead by a few steps. The stones of Australians (and

Cubans?) might be the lightest by the time we reach 2020. The importance of looking at the situation in Cuba is neatly argued for by Jerry Spiegel and Annalee Yassi, in *Lessons from the margins of globalization: appreciating the Cuban Health Paradox*, wherein the following quotations aid to strike the match in vigorous fashion:

"Despite widespread recognition of Cuba's achievements in producing excellent health outcomes out of proportion for such a poor country, the world scientific and public policy communities are scarcely learning what they should from this experience."
[Cuba is currently ranked between 63rd and 71st in the world in terms of nominal GDP, depending on which global authority does the ranking; Rodriguez, Lopez and Choonara (2008), in *Child health in Cuba*, says Cuba is the 120th wealthiest country in the world]

"Cuba's experience presents nothing less than a fundamental paradox or challenge to the assumption that generating wealth is the fundamental precondition for improving health – which may itself explain the wish by some to ignore, contest, or even hide this country's achievements."

What makes the Cuban model of health so attractive, at least from political and economic points of view? Well, Cubans prove that you don't have to be rich to be healthy. Point taken. Repeat: *you don't have to be rich to be healthy*. Repeat again, until it creates that light bulb-feeling. Doctors are not paid much in Cuba, unlike in other countries, but the Cubans have shown that the right kinds of investment in education alongside health can significantly lower the prevalence rates – or even eradicate – the existence of serious diseases and conditions such as polio, neonatal tetanus, diphtheria, measles, whooping cough, rubella and hepatitis-B. Cuba boasts the lowest U5MR (under-5 (child) mortality rate) and the greatest reduction in U5MR in Latin America and the Carribean, and competes directly with the USA and the

UK (two of the top ten richest nations on earth) with respect to this indicator. How were the Cuban government and people able to do this? According to two or three of the very few internationally accepted publications (note that there exists sanctions against academic material published by Cuban authors), the success of the Cuban healthcare system is attributed to its basic functional unit, the municipal polyclinic. These integrative polyclinics were created already in 1963 and served as centers created specifically for ambulatory care; they were specifically charged "with directing all health activities aimed at persons or the environment within their jurisdiction" (Novas & Fernandez Sacasas, 1989, *Revista Cubana de Medicina General Integral*, Vol. 5, No. 4, pp. 556-564). During the early 1980s Fidel Castro Ruz initiated the establishment of the family doctor specialty, and subsequently the formation of family doctor-and-nurse teams which ultimately raised the effectiveness of the healthcare approach to monumental levels that remain the envy of many healthcare authorities from around the globe. To achieve this, each polyclinic was subdivided in order to extend the reach of the healthcare platform: small primary centers called *consultario* were located across Cuba and each is staff by a family doctor and a nurse; both the family doctor and the nurse live next to or very close to the consultario. In 2008 there were more than 15 000 of these consultarios across Cuba and each served between 120 and 160 families. Between 30 and 40 family doctors grouped under one polyclinic; the polyclinic is empowered to offer a standard variety of specialist options, including paediatrics, dentistry, social work, physiotherapy and clinical psychology (larger polyclinics can offer a wider variety of other specialties). In this way, any child or adult in any location across Cuba can have weekly access to specialist services, provided by government. If it were possible to substitute the name of any other country for Cuba in the preceding sentence, the healthcare world would have achieved one of its most important goals in the 21st century. This is exactly the stated goal to which we must align our efforts in order to provide *Healthcare for ALL!*

Cuba has indeed proved that it is possible to achieve a better state of health even in the face of such an ubiquitous spread of poverty – we cannot continue to believe the contrary notion of it being impossible to be healthy while being poorer (by whatever standards you choose to measure). Evidence refutes belief. How is it that a poorer country is better able to lighten its stone than what most of the richer countries are able to do theirs? If, for once, you can concede that healthcare systems in the richer countries are not put in place primarily to address issues of health, then you can certainly comprehend how we can move closer to achieving what would have seemed to be impossible up till now. The tipping point is that each individual can contribute by realizing the self-responsibility toward individual health. According to the most noble-hearted Paul Freire, democracy is not an individual property (cf. *Teachers as cultural workers*), but healthcare is – this is worth reemphasizing a few thousand times: if you take your own health more seriously, not only in word and intention, but more so in deed and action, then you are already making the world a much better place. Healthcare is personal; it's about you: *ALL about YOU*. There should be no democracy in your claim to take responsibility for your own health; you should be totally in charge of your own health. However the government decides to tackle its claim of responsibility for health of its respective peoples – which could be democratic, socialistic, capitalistic, communistic or whatever other -*tic* you can think of – it's up to the respective government. However, it's not up to your government to take responsibility for your health. It never was, and never should be.

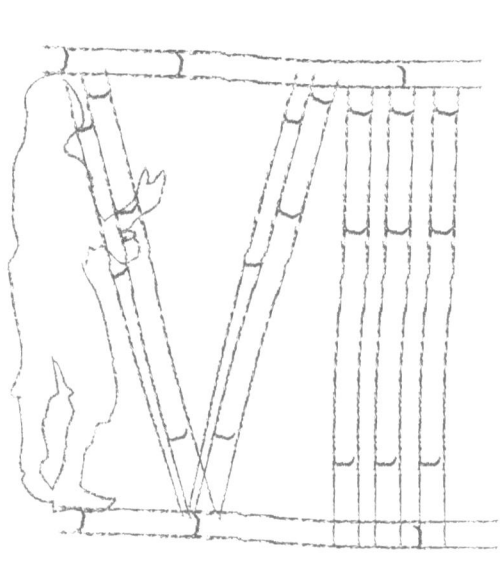

"The truth is, unless you let go, unless you forgive yourself, unless you forgive the situation, unless you realize that the situation is over, you cannot move forward."

Steve Maraboli

.

eighth RELEASE

Talking about heavy stones can often bring about the dreadful feeling of a pervasive heaviness that sucks into it all of the surroundings; a heaviness that drains you from all reserves of physical or psycho-spiritual energy. Granted, we need to be aware of our situation, we must indeed contemplate each of the factors into its simplest manifestations and bring to our conscious awareness as much as is needed to overcome the effects that we've allowed onto or into ourselves till now; we must own the problem before we can correct for the course of action we are to take from here, but, alas, we need to exhale those feelings and all the associated negativity; it needs to pass through us, we need to feel it! Then we must let go – all the negative associations that came with the discussion of health, healthcare financing or other pressing issues in the domain of health or disease. We must clear the air in our minds – we must start looking ahead to something that will be much more energy efficient.

There needs to a release, a dedicated effort to leave to the wind those things that will not nccd to bog us down any longer. A vent is needed; it is a natural requirement. The wider the opening, the less pressure there will be; the more we can heal. However, we cannot lose ourselves when allowing the release; we retain our self-respect; that dignified composure – regardless of age, there is no shame in unlearning and relearning concepts in life that will benefit us and those we cherish. To heal within we need to acknowledge our individual parts to play; only from here can we positively aspire to achieve greater heights of individual health, and subsequently, healthier environments and societies.

Do we know what to release, how to release it and when to do so? We're in the process of changing how we understand our health, our healthcare responsibility and our individualized claim to better health. However, in admitting that we need to change something also implies that whatever we tried before didn't work out as well as we wanted it to. This is the part that brings pain: we invested money – we believed we did the right thing, we built our lives around those beliefs, and we made sure that everyone in our households aligns with it – even at the expense of balanced interpersonal relationships. For sure, we would not need to change things if things were going very well as they are, would we? Issues at stake would be healthcare insurance and access to it (or the lack thereof), choice of family health professionals, locations of treatment, willingness to participate in activities geared toward improving our health, choice of schools for our children, and so forth. Despite the best of decisions that were made, things still happened as they have been doing, dragging most of the progressive world into pits of uncertainty.

The pain, of knowing now we could have done something different to affect different outcomes, is a heaviness to bear. It developed into a pain as we started understanding that events in our everyday healthcare lives are not happening toward the best or most progressive of outcomes, due to a wide range of possible reasons most notably including how we are supported by our governments and public programs in achieving our stated goals of health. There is pain in the error of the past. This we must acknowledge. Something failed, we failed, the government failed, *this* failed, and *that* failed. The list is endless, and growing. Failure is painful. This is the pain that needs to be released. As the pain is released we also need to let those emotions go – those emotions that expressed themselves within us, those emotions that became part of our psyche, our everyday reference to matters of personal effect. Some major part of our personalities is attributed to the experiences we go through; if these experiences were mostly negative, it is not surprising that our personality traits include major expressions of depression, anxiety, fear or hatred. Knowing this can cause pain, or emotional turbulence (to borrow from Dr. Deepak Chopra), and this is the type of turbulence that can cause further destruction on our paths to happiness. Reading about it can be painful; thinking about it can evoke stronger emotions. We must want to experience these emotions, but only for the sake of having experienced them so that we can release them. We must allow the emotion to be, in itself, for itself; else we can never claim to having overcome it. Acknowledge this pain, the pain of the past, and let it be. Just let it be. A new wave of experience is approaching, something radically different, and to be best prepared for a different type of life, we need to release the pain of the past.

Not everything we did in the past was wrong – of course not. We very rarely always do the wrong things, but we also very rarely always do the right things (assuming that we generally adopt a right-versus-wrong approach to life). It is perhaps preferable to think along the lines of what is appropriate to do, set against actions not deemed as appropriate; meaning that it may be more worthwhile to judge our efforts by how appropriate our actions and decisions are as opposed to how right or how wrong they are. Every situation is embedded in a context, and every decision must be based on the merits of that particular context. Collectively, the total sum of outcomes, today, is as a direct or indirect consequence of all the smallest of individual actions undertaken on a daily basis, over a period of time. This roughly translates to the notion that the 2008 economic crisis can be blamed to every individual on the planet who lived up to that moment in time (for simplicity let's narrow it down to the times from after the Great Depression to the 2008 calendar); this is evident that the whole world was hugely affected by the events surrounding the great loss of monetary wealth and livelihoods. It would be senseless to single out one individual; hence the term global catastrophe. From the highest (in stature) to the lowest were affected, some more than others; in the end, something major happened in the world that made us all feel the acute level of interconnectedness that we so often dismiss. The world of right and wrong becomes a jungle of uncertainty – how can it be right that a few selected people could be responsible for an event that shook the psyche of the world? Well, how can it be wrong? We allowed it to happen. The fact that it was allowed makes us part of it.

Yes, *we allowed it* - each one of us, every able adult in this world. Especially those who felt it were not their prerogative to meddle in the affairs of those in charge. By stepping away from the hot seat we left it to those few to get the best of what the trading world had to offer, unchecked. We forsook our responsibility to our well-being, we neglected our roles as guardians of our own health, a role that otherwisely required due diligence. True citizenship is a very intricate matter requiring a very noble sense of entitlement and appropriate action. What we did wrong is that we did not inform ourselves as best as we could have; we allowed ourselves to be led astray by those with some form of perceived superiority. This is a severe punishment for laziness, a mental laziness that translated into an absent form of citizenship. We were lazy, we were ignorant, and we were not as diligent as we could have been. We were all these things at some point in time; we are not totally wrong or right, or totally blind, or totally left out in the cold. There is pain in this level of awareness, a fact that is completely rational and totally allowable. Now, we release that pain, and we next look to understand how we can let that pain go without losing that core sense of true self.

Without the necessary focus on any specific, chronological sequence, the most appropriate actions for a rational and dignified release would be one or a selection of the following: (1) accept what has been (in the past) and acknowledge your part in creating the type of life you are currently living, and become fully aware that if anything were ever going to be better, it starts with you making the choice to do things differently, and to make the appropriate changes to your life that can effect more positive and progressive outcomes; (2) accept that it is necessary to be angry, upset, demoralized, or experience any other negative emotion with regards to your current state of health and quality of life – once you allow these emotions, it would be extremely helpful to express them (write them, sing them, talk to your friends or family members about them, etc.); (3) accept that you do not have to feel embarrassed by mistakes you made because you did not know about things that could have helped you to make better decisions; (4) even if you have been making poor decisions despite possessing better knowledge, accept that things are not cast in stone and that you can overturn those decisions once you concentrate your efforts towards a more individual approach to your healthcare and the health of those entrusted to you; (5) make the decision to forgive whomever you previously would call "the enemy" (even and especially if it is yourself), commit to stop blaming the government, your neighbors or any other entity – they cannot be held responsible for your health because you can be your own worst enemy when it comes to matters of health (not everyone understands the concept of forgiveness; in this case, grant amnesty to those you think are to be blamed; when amnesty is granted, the focus entirely shifts to the present and on what your next step in life will be in terms of your well-being and your health); (6) accept that it is time to release all of the past; accept to leave things of the past to the past; do not reserve any emotional space for those things in the now or any possible conjectured future; (7) let it be; as things were, let them be. Change what you need to change, do it now; start right this very moment. It is surely the only way to move ahead, progressively so. Breathe it out, open your vents and give it to the sky.

When is the best time to release? _Now_ is the best time – as we just entered a new year in the aftermath of a grueling 2013 – one year after the supposed 'end-of-the-world year'. Well, the world may not have ended, but something big is definitely coming to an end. Medical dominance, as some of us academics may call it (cf. Mark Bahnisch and his work on "Medical Dominance"), is coming to an end. Societies across the globe have been medicalized, and the world of occupations was dominated by the medical profession. Healthcare regimes are opting towards privatization – medical doctors are finally set into the world of business, where the best service provider will have to provide best service in order to be profitable. As the individual consumer you will have more options and better service; your government and your healthcare providers will enforce these options and services. It's a movement that already gained a huge following in the

1990s, but only now does it have the necessary impetus to enforce a global force of action that will finally break the stronghold of the select few who stood by silently as we went ahead in supporting a growing medical industry at the expense of our health. All of the recent events in our collective history points to the fact that something major is happening in the world – this cannot be refuted. It is manifested naturally as well as within the minds of those who contribute to the philosophical and spiritual development of mankind. There is major resistance against ideas of mind manifesting as natural events, but even with this type of resistance, the power of an individual mind is rising up on a more regular basis. In knowing this it is indeed noteworthy to point out that each reader can be empowered to make most meaningful changes in the approach to healthcare, far beyond anything that has happened during the previous fifty years. It could be overwhelming to realize that a different approach to health, by the individual, can lead to the establishment of a whole new regime of healthcare and fundamental changes in the medical world, in ways that were never seen since the days of the invention of pasteurization.

The fact that you have this book in your hands, or these words on your LCD screen, is testament to the fact that change is imminent, that you want a different set of outcomes to what you may have had before; or that you'd also like to see a more progressive world in which people are actually healthier. It cannot be denied, as much as I could not stop myself from writing this book (even in the face of career suicide). We need to change the way in which we think about our health, and we now have an idea of what type of change is needed. The vital next step would be to acknowledge the need for change and accept to be part of it. Change is inevitable, as inevitable as the continued suffering that will result if no change will occur.

.

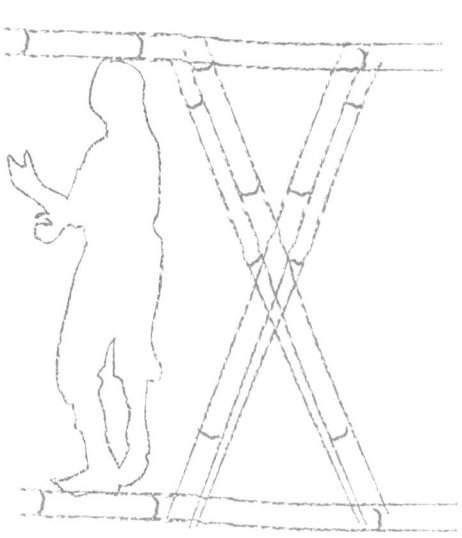

"We should remember
that just as a positive outlook on life
can promote good health,
so can everyday acts of kindness."

Hillary Rodham Clinton

ninth ACT

Once the philosophy behind a novel or freshened approach has been elucidated, how does one proceed to action? One typically starts to talk about things in a more pragmatic sense – what can be done, by you or me, to act in ways that correspond to the new or changed ways of thinking we have formulated in our minds? A series of suggested actions are provided, as a preliminary guide, to be followed as the reader deems fit. It is not a decisive guide; I make no claims to be an authoritative voice – these steps are synthesized and formulated from my personal and work-based experiences in different healthcare environments. Academics involved in medical education seem to like the terms 'quality control' and 'participatory action research'; from these types of research-based experiences companies and leaders of institutions can gauge how effective their programs are. Considering that this book, in context of the publication series Chaos in Medicine™, is a first to view the medical profession from the stated point of view as explained in earlier chapters (Volume 1), we can safely ascertain that this collection of chapters should serve as a conversation starter. This conversation would be the base conversation that takes us into what we can call *The New Dispensation of Health(care)*. From this point of view, the steps suggested below must be analyzed, criticized and commented upon, for only through proper public discourse can we carve out more progressive pathways as we head into the unknown future. The author here makes a best effort to write the steps in a logical order, suggesting some form of chronological sequence, but with added insights from other readers and commentators we can continue to refine and combine our different understandings of this complex phenomenon until we have more concrete plans that will take us to the actions of tomorrow from which a better state of health will emerge.

Assessing your situation

Look around you with the purpose of assessing your situation. The question that needs answering is "*how well am I disposed with regards to achieving a very good state of health, for myself, and for my family*"? If you are reading this book as a team (which is recommended), then substitute the singular for a plural pronoun; henceforth the pronouns "you" or "we" can refer to either a single individual or a family. How healthy are you? With what you have to your disposal, as it fits your lifestyle and your budget, in what condition are you? As mentioned before (as with the example using an online search engine to look up health needs), this is a multi-layered question. The assessment is primarily aimed at waking up (if sleeping) or reinforcing (if already active) a certain level of conscientiousness with regards to how you really are (or how I am, if the question is addressed to me), as if we'd be really, really honest if someone were to ask, "Hey, how (healthy) are you?"

Are you in a panicky state, forever fretting about things? Where does it come from and why does it happen? Are you generally nervous, making many mistakes in your daily interactions with people, also 'missing out' on a lot of things because of your constant, nervous agitation? Are you excessively happy, never letting anyone know how much pain you're hiding? Is there something physically wrong when you eat, sleep, walk or run? Perhaps when you're reading, or try to read, you fall asleep every time, feeling so tired that you dread having to read at all. Are you super-charged all the time, or do you feel like sitting whenever you need to stand? Do you have illnesses that only you really know you have but you're afraid to have an official diagnoses; do you have a drug habit that only you and some mysterious, clandestine friends know about? What about your appetite for food, for adventure, for living, for being ambitious? Do you have friends, good conversations, regular sex, or other religious or spiritual interests that add positive value to your life? Does life appeal to you, or do you rather prefer to stay away from anything alive? Do you fear relationships so much that you rather stay alone? If in a relationship with another (marriage, co-habitation, or otherwise), do you give of your best to that person or the relationship, also in terms of your physical state and abilities? Do you have a good job, are you making good money (in the legal sense of the word), or does your happiness or health depend on your job? Are you fat, thin, obese, anorexic, bulimic, slightly overweight or any other way of being that makes you feel terribly afraid of being around other people? Does your skin itch all the time and are you afraid to touch other people? Do you live a happy life and feel that you are totally content and in need of none? There are so many questions, and perhaps it may come as a shock when looking at your life from all the different angles as represented by these questions, but in each of them there's a direct link to your state of health. Yes, your state of health determines how you deal with life, or how you are able to deal with it. Therefore, quite logically, it follows that you need to assess this thing about yourself: you must know how healthy you are, in every sense of the word and within the many different manifestations thereof.

Having a family, of course, adds another few dimensions to this assessment. Children grow quickly and parents must know how best to serve their children during these periods of quick growth. Teaching children about health requires that parents are themselves the experts on health, seen from a child's point of view; so, how can we as parents be so resistant to learning more about healthcare provision when it is required that we equip ourselves with some of the knowledge of experts, at least for the sake of managing our households? You cannot refer your child to a doctor every time you have problems with health. This sounds far-fetched, perhaps, but so many people are dependent on an official medical opinion before they are moved toward a definitive action of some kind. Where does this reliance on official diagnoses come from? For one of a few strong possibilities, it probably comes from parents who did not take it within the parental stride to teach a few good basics that would have rendered the growing adult less dependent on the official healthcare system.

Again, who knows more about the child other than the child itself? Of course, the parent does. It's not the doctor who knows more about your child. Your child grew up under your guise and no one is qualified to take better care of your child. Well, no one should be, else you should not have children – this issue repeatedly surfaces in contemporary literature in the form of a common question, "*Why do people have more children if they're not willing to fully immerse in taking the appropriate actions of caring that are needed for raising healthy individuals?*" This issue can be fully addressed elsewhere, but what is important to consider is that we need to become more aware of our responsibilities toward our children. You may wonder why it is so. Think about it in this way: if you accept that your personality and stature in life are constructs heavily affected by your environment, then where does your healthcare begin? It begins at your birth, a time when you cannot accept responsibility for it. Who accepts this responsibility? Your parents, of course. Your healthcare started with your parents (or legal guardians) and they, initially, determine much of how you adapt to the environment (let's use the generic term *parents* to include those in your life who accepted primary responsibility for your well-being, on your behalf, while you were not able to do so).

Now, when did your healthcare become your responsibility? Well, this would be the next step in our assessment of where we are. When did we really start taking responsibility for our health? From our fresher perspective, we can already assume this responsibility as soon as we are able to find our way in the world. If you can teach a three year-old boy to protect himself from a kettle with boiling water, then of course you can start teaching him about healthcare. Into the future, though, you do not teach your child to be dependent on any medical service outside your home. Medical services, as an industry of service professionals, will be there to assist, not to take responsibility. Are your children aware of their responsibilities toward themselves, first and foremost? If this is not met with a nod, then the work has to start from exactly this point – proving that this assessment would then already have yielded significant findings. It is the parent who must teach the child about the self-responsibility to health. Should the parent fail in this regard, the child grows up to become dependent on other possible sources for advice and guidance on matters of health. Should you fail as a parent in the duty to teach these basics to your child, it becomes a burden on other

126

parents and adults to try to build such a foundation in your child's life. Once the child reaches a certain age (say, for example, six or seven years old), it becomes too difficult to teach new habits and sometimes it will already be impossible to affect a certain level of self-caring in the growing individual.

Gather those around you; start this conversation and continue it for a few days, over weeks, till everyone understands the notion that talking about health is an everyday matter, not to be hidden; pride, silliness or other behavioral notions commonly prevent necessary disclosure. In fact, this type of non-disclosure is so common and forms the crux of many story lines of modern-day TV dramas and series involving parents and children in everyday situations. This book is not a step-by-step guide to parenting, but the insistence here is on developing a certain kind of habit by which a family will benefit, for obvious reasons. Assessing the state of health for your household is a responsibility of those who head the house, but it is not the responsibility of those who head the house to keep everyone healthy. Those (adults) in charge can learn how to assist and provide guidance, by being more aware of what exactly is happening when room doors are closed (that normally hide the coughing, sneezing, silent ailing or other types of symptoms that might have exposed the illness or disease). If things go really well with this kind of assessment, we'd be able to identify – as well as diagnose and treat – more of the prevalent diseases, imbalances and illnesses with which our families are so commonly afflicted.

Some academics may recognize the underlying theme in this advancement of admonishment, which pivots around the issue of the sick role as medical literature has coined it. Yes, strangely so, academics have arrived at the point (many years ago, in fact) of understanding that some people enjoy being sick. It sounds weird – "how can you enjoy being sick?" you may wonder – but patients have been subjected to many kinds of studies that focus on patient behavior in medical settings or patient homes. There are huge chunks of observation-based data that show that people abuse their rights to being labeled sick, which affect most of the other aspects of their social and working lives. How could it be that a progressive society is composed of a majority of people who enjoy being sick? Could you apply the term "progressive" to them, or would you rather say "sick society"? This is what I am advocating against – we cannot continually raise our children to the point where they'd do anything (even play sick) to benefit more from an insurance or healthcare advantage by a chosen service provider. It is not okay to be sick – only mentally handicapped or spiritually depressed people are arguably justified to enjoy sickness; the very nature of this darkened psyche needs to illuminated upon. We should stop playing sick and we should start admitting (at least to those in our households) when our health is not as good as it could be; and we should start living a type of life where we celebrate our health by living better lives in healthier environments. As said before, this type of assessment runs across all aspects of our lives and should be conducted under the frame of mind that seeks to make things healthier and better.

Surveying your immediate surroundings

This being a pen-and-paper task, tied with some serious contemplation, the next step in the series of steps toward acting in more progressive and constructive sets of behavior lies in making your own resource survey, i.e. taking stock of what you have around you and, perhaps more importantly, what you do not have around you. This activity will allow you to become more familiar with those services and human resource potential in your immediate residential area that you have to your disposal, or that you didn't know you have, or that you thought you had but don't actually have. In some cases, for the sake of health, you will not only be looking for things traditionally labeled as healthcare resources. A fire station can also be a health resource – firefighters are trained in basic health and first aid, and can often show you the right direction toward finding more appropriate healthcare expertise. The library would also be an excellent health resource. Yes, resist as much as you want, but doctors and nurses read too; some of their reference books can be found in your very own backyard library.

I mention the word resource, mainly attempting to convey the idea that we have the duty toward ourselves in knowing a bit more than we currently do. It's the information age and there's not much we can do about the fact that it's so much easier than before to access certain types of information. We also cannot suddenly jump up and create the sort of plans that turn us into non-accredited pseudo-professionals, like some fugitives do; we should use these resources to aid in our own knowledge of ourselves to the point where we are better equipped to care for ourselves. We can learn to have healthier hair or skin, healthier eating or drinking habits, or healthier interpersonal relationships. At either the simplest or deeper levels of health manifestation, these things correlate directly with our state of health. Most knowledge pertaining to these aspects of our lives can be found in a library (whether online or in physical paper format), and if we're open to it, we can actually create a health revolution around the world where people are more open to take the matter of health into their own hands – by being more dependent on their own individual effort than on the expertise of someone who might or might not understand how best to advise on individual health – for the sake of showing the best way to health instead of basing the decision on profit margins.

Walk around your neighborhood. Make a list of buildings with the purpose of each. What proportion of resources is allocated to health, let's say *neighborhood health*, to give it a name? Then think about how easy or difficult it is for you to access those places. Are they open to general enquiries – do the attending workers in those places allow members from the public to seek for help, do they offer help when such requests are made? Can my neighborhood be healthier by way of how these resources are allocated? Can my family use these resources and places as stepping stones toward achieving better family health? If there would be resources, do I have the liberty to make my own approach in seeking advice and services (here we must pause, this is often the most difficult part for many people)? Do I currently have the habit of seeking advice and services from these places? If I (the adult) were able to obtain the services or advice from these resources and those people in charge of it, would the rest of my family know how to achieve such a simple task? In one household, we should all know how to do these things even if the real-life emergency never occurs. Health-related emergencies happen often enough for most people to use these skills only once or twice in, for argument's sake, a decade – but it is of vital importance that everyone in the house knows exactly how to access the avenues of help and assistance when they're needed. This type of attitude would signify a healthier outlook on life and underscores the importance of having to take the responsibility of our own health unto ourselves, first and foremost.

Next, consider and note whether you have access (in your own neighborhood, of course) to any of the following: gyms, clinics, hospitals, any place dispensing medicine or medical advice, schools (and school facilities), beauty or lifestyle treatment business, shopping malls with these services, alternative healing practices (remember, these are not from the devil; many of the alternative approaches to mainstream medicine has proven much more effective than corresponding western treatments), geriatric facilities, or any other places associated with these resources.

Take a community newspaper and look for ads that contain information that show you how to access these place or their services. Many people browse through newspaper pages and selectively ignore this type of information – the decision to ignore could be based on a range of possible reasons. There are also possibilities of people ignoring or denying the use of these services due to financial considerations. To the contrary, however, one can benefit from knowing what exactly is offered by all these types of institutions or businesses because knowledge of peoples' main business often takes you to understanding what they do on the social side of life that perhaps help them (or their businesses) with staying healthier. Of course, our streets and neighborhoods at times are filled with strange characters, but beyond all that you may find networks of individuals that work hard at keeping healthier despite the negative things they may be surrounded with.

We are humans and we tend to socialize; there is no harm in stepping out of your comfort zone to appropriate the type of communal coexistence that could remarkably improve the odds of you and your family attaining better health amidst limited resource availability. In today's climate of crushing economic vicissitudes, one should not despair at the prospect of sharing resources. Even if it may appear counterintuitive, resistance against sharing will continue to make us sicker, especially if we accept that health is an all-encompassing construct within our lives. Although this specific exercise started with noting the number of health-related resources you have to your disposal, we now end up with contemplating how best to share what we have. Yet again, by looking at how children tend to do things when they are still in their free stages of expression, we can learn valuable lessons. Sharing brings joy more than what it creates sadness; it enhances human relationships rather than forging a perpetual divide between different kinds of people; and it opens up many more doors toward a better world as opposed to keeping those doors close in the face of any resistance to sharing.

We can and therefore should share the resources. In your neighborhood, what are the resources that can be shared more? Have you used these resources, or do you rather prefer to stay locked up in your own home and your own, perfectly warm comfort zone, where the lack of human interaction could actually damage your chances to a better state of health? It is worth a consideration. On the other hand, diseases and germs are things we do not want to share; however, the more you stay locked up the least able your defenses against very simple germs will be, the higher your need for insurance will become and the less likely you'll be able to form what was previously known as *normal relationships with everyday people.* Diseases and germs have always been part of society; it is not always known how people get sick even despite rigorous anti-germ lifestyles, but a healthier life is not lived in total isolation of the world. It never was thus and never should be.

Even within the same neighborhood some families are healthier than others. Unpacking the many reasons behind this is the matter of postgraduate sociology research, but as a hypothesis it could be ventured that in a significant number of cases the main differences in the outcomes of health states for different families lay within the knowledge of which resources are used and how often these resources are accessed[1]. After your own penciling of the list of resources and services, it would be worth comparing your list to those of your friends or acquaintances. The feedback and inherent discussions should provide meaningful insights that could just add that extra little bit of light on the road ahead. For this, blogging and texting could be useful avenues of action. I am willing to bet that most of us will be alarmed as to what exactly we have within a one or two-mile radius away from us. If you're willing to put some of your retaliations aside (e.g. religion, ethnicity, race), you might actually be rather surprised to learn quite a bit of handy things from those people around you. You may even have some resources at your disposal that others could never have known of. We could call it "sharing-health", where we could be open to sharing things again as people did many,

---

[1] Some would conveniently assert that some families are healthier because they have more money or wealth and it is exactly this conjecture that needs to be challenged. Attached to this issue is the philosophical notion of having the right to claim that one person is *healthier* than another; we have *indices* of health or health outcomes, but what does it mean to be *healthier*?

many years ago; the sharing aspect will spill over into so many other aspects of our lives, it could potentially just change you for the better, once and for all. I am once again reminded of the book *The Happiness Project* in which the author made a very committed effort to showing how sharing brings so much real value back to normal, everyday lives.

Getting involved: primary care and community health

Find out what primary healthcare is, the scope of it and how you can become better equipped for dealing with issues of health at your home or in the confines of your family or immediate circle of influence. This is the time where you can learn to visit the doctor or nurse at your local clinic for a reason other than collecting medicine or treatment. I know; this might induce a shock, not only to you, but to those nurses, doctors and other healthcare personnel in the setting. Imagine the feedback to the facility manager, "the patient is visiting us for purposes of learning about how to take better care of the family or an individual – she's not here for a treatment". With a list of questions and readiness for receiving a whole range of care-related answers, each one of us can change how the healthcare system (as provided by the state) can be of benefit to us. Of course, the government is not going to send your medicine by mail and the pharmacist will certainly not drive around in a delivery pick-up to drop off drugs, but there are some things that you can definitely do that will help yourself and your family to a state of mind that can lead to a happier and healthier state of being. The pencil-and-paper method is just one way – you can substitute it for an iPad if you like – but the gist of the whole idea is for you to become more proactive in assessing and dealing with your health.

***

We don't like this word – proactive – and it has been shown many times over. I bet this sentence containing the word proactive will be deleted in future editions of writers whose paraphrasing of this text might help to get stubborn consumerist mindsets to eventually participate in more proactive campaigns, but the perpetual insistence on the part of the author (for the reader to be more proactive) is based on solid evidence that proactivity by large masses of people within a population can surely calm the swelling tides of deteriorated health. In fact, greater cooperation and proactivity directly decreases the prevalence of a number of known illnesses or diseases, even by people living in very poor communities. It has been proven, so if you state that it is not true then your argument has just been shown to have no leg to stand on; in other words, we have just amputated the leg of ignorance and now you can be open to the one thing that might just pull you out from under those thick layers of denial: primary healthcare and how it builds community health.

You need to get out. Out in the open – where other people are using the same resources as you. No matter who you are, you must share. There are seven billion living human beings on earth (and counting...); the requirement for sharing is becoming an absolute necessity. If you can comfortably stab this notion to pieces it means that you are one of a very few elite individuals who don't need to move in public space at all. This book is probably not meant for those elite individuals, but the rest of us are definitely included in this space bracket. Primary healthcare is healthcare at its most basic level. The idea of primary health is not new, but having it at the heart of medical practice (in the western world, at least) is a very new thing. Anything primary, to most people, would mean of highest importance, but to the top-notch medical professionals it actually means of least importance. Except for those who supply the instruments and medicine for primary care, there's not much profit involved in primary healthcare and, guess what, it's the reason why we are not as well-served as we ought to be. There are many so-called experts out there who can tell you volumes of encyclopedic knowledge about primary care, but we don't really know so much about it as we would like to. Primary healthcare is about individual healthcare, if taken down to the core, and the medical fraternity has only just begun to investigate and understand how everyday life impacts on primary health.

The surprise element here is that you know more than your doctor about your primary health. I bet you do and I'd conduct research to prove the point. You live in the street far away from the academic hospital and you are the only one who can give a really accurate account of how the environment impacts on you. By the time you enter the medical practice, you are so far removed from your normal environment that the doctor or nurse cannot possibly know, with any absolute amount of certainty, how best to treat you, regardless of how well-qualified they are. (We are, of course, assuming that you are of sound mind and rational conduct; for people not within this classification, the issue of healthcare becomes a bit murkier). For this reason, you ought to invest in your own study and understanding of primary healthcare and how it pertains to your life and surroundings. Primary healthcare is no longer something that only the experts should know about. That would be traditional thinking and also exactly the reason why the medical profession could assert its total dominance over the public sector – people conveniently left it to the professionals to make decisions on behalf of patients when most of those decisions were better made if the patients were more aware of what has been happening in their own lives. If you have a habit of finding information and this habit is inculcated from a very early age, then of course your life and decisions as an adult will be different; you might better learn the art of balancing a reactive mindset with a proactive approach. I agree; it's a pity and shame that we were not always led to the right doors when we were younger; however, now that we know of better, we can start affecting the necessary change. *"Be the change that you wish to see in the world"*. Become the paragon of health you want the world to be.

Community health is a mathematical extension of primary health. If more people take their individual primary health more seriously, it follows naturally (even at exponential rates) that communities will also improve their respective health indicators. Being part of a community is what ultimately makes us happy; if the community is healthy it will also be happy. Unhealthy communities allow unhealthy and other ungodly or unsightly profanities; we would therefore love to see this change. We talk about it all the time; we reflect on how nice it was back then – but how is it that we remain unmoved by how things have turned out, especially during times of economic hardship? We cannot be unmoved; that is impossible. My brain cannot fathom the immovability in people who falsely declare their passion and interest for making things better. Yes, we have problems mixing with people from different backgrounds, ethnicities and origins, but we cannot continue holding these up as blinker pads against our faces; we need to let it go; somehow, somewhere. The world has changed dramatically over the last twenty years; the terms globalization and multi-cultural exchange strike us with fear and loathsomeness. Our governments are trying hard to cooperate for economic gain, but on the street level we continue to insist on the ways that will make us happy, not always having regard for the needs of others of differential origins. Woven into all these dynamics is the issue of our health; if we need to learn to share for the sake of our health within the community we're presently part of, then we'd better get it on with (as the expression goes) and start changing our attitudes. No-one likes to be wrong, but your ways and views are not always right, or the most correct.

Sharing is the buzz-word; it is the concept for the 21st century, and the lack of it is definitely one major obstacle in a growing list of obstacles to achieving better health. Community health cannot be about one person. Community health is important and it should be an important consideration for every member that makes up that community. You are part of a community whether you like it or not, especially when you buy groceries at the community supermarket, when your child attends the community school or college, when you rush a sick child to the community hospital or clinic, or when you need a plumber after midnight and the janitor happens to be from another ethnicity but knows the one plumber closest to where you live. It would probably be better to say that the most debilitating disease humans brought with them from the 20th century is alienation and chronic, racial hypersensitivity. Once we find ways to combat these diseases, we'd probably have a miraculous wave of increased healthcare indicators. Sufficiently strong emotions (hatred, anxiety, fear), for a long enough time, can cause illness. Community health entails a holistic approach to healing, and this century will witness how being one's being nicer to a neighbor can decrease the prevalence of hypertension, high blood pressure and even liver cirrhosis. If your health is really that important to you, you will consider accepting your community, especially if you think that a nicer community will allow you to be nicer person. Strangely, it is you who'd have to be nice first, before the community can become nicer. Nicer communities will have healthier people, and healthier people will create nicer communities.

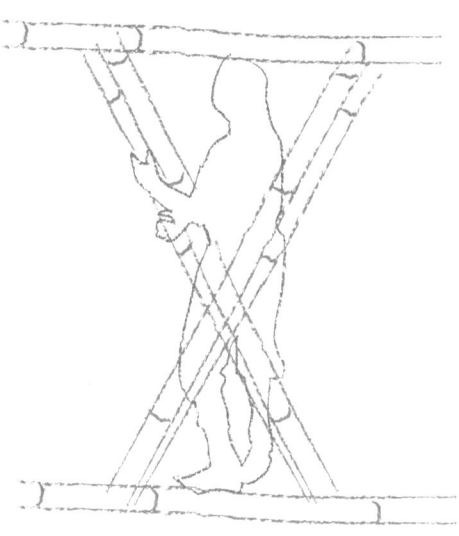

"That which is like unto itself is drawn."

from the Law of Attraction

tenth COMMANDMENT OF HEALTH

Awareness of the law of healing places on us the responsibility of knowing about the balance of energies within and around us; with a delicate balance we are healthy, an imbalance renders us uncomfortable, sick or diseased. As a command from nature, thus, we ought to take priority into matters of our healthcare. This commandment thus speaks from the very nature of which we are part and it speaks to us in the sternest of tones, a desperate call to arms for we have allowed ourselves to be driven toward the most depressed state of consciousness since the beginning of (human) time. What we have allowed up till now is not easily undone; before we move ahead we need to acknowledge the depth and gravity of our true contexts, not cloaked in poetic verse that allows us to proportion any blame or responsibility to another entity but self. It is by looking within that we find what we can do to change what lives on the outside; the inner reflects in the outer, the outer depends on the inner voice that constantly seeks to place itself within hearing range of the soul who wishes to listen. Health is an important matter and we cannot forsake our individual responsibilities toward ourselves and those entrusted to us, hoping that, someday, someone or something will come to rescue us. We are capable of making the appropriate choices and we would be best served if we stop waiting for a better time in the future to change what we need to change this very instant.

We could, of course, exercise our rights and refuse to budge; in fact, if you decide to conveniently forget what has been written (that which was wrote was writ in the mind of illuminating a dark, mysterious horse) then it doesn't even reach the stage of exercising a right. No single person has the right to force a different viewpoint onto anyone else. The author writes with the intent of sharing an idea, starting a conversation or to convey a certain impression. The reader is under no obligation to respond. Knowing this, why do people write, why has this book been written, just why would one person spend more than a decade thinking about writing a book when he knows the reader will just plainly ignore any of the insights and impressions? Well, just as you feel you have the democratic right to your viewpoint, the author, as a medical researcher, has the right to share knowledge regarding the observations while interacting with people just like you. This would almost be like "show & tell" with you not really caring about who listens or not. My *show & tell* comes with a slight difference: I have sympathy pains when I see people in pain. It was my job to conduct medical education research; it was not my job to observe the pain of patients. The more I moved through different medical settings the more I realized they all have something in common; something much more profound than the medical education research I was conducting with medical students. I realized that people enter medical settings with loads of pain – psychological pain, spiritual neglect or emptiness, mental depression, anger, hatred, indifference and even pain associated with suicidal notions. I felt these energies and I, too, relate to some of those feelings and emotions. Medical science does it's best to stay away from the issue of feelings and emotions; it does very little to assuage the concerns of those it swears to serve. There are many concerns of health that are not addressed; by professional and other legal laws these concerns cannot be voiced, and when they are stifled in this manner, they create disease and illness.

This is what I noticed – these are the similarities between settings I observed and noted. And I've seen the reader there, too. I disguised myself as not being part of the setting, but I too had to swim in the sea of all interacting human emotions. It's a spiritual nightmare and the world needs a waking up. If you went to a medical setting over the last twenty years, I've seen you. I've seen you a million times over in the persona of someone else. We are not as different as we like to believe through our constant language or culture-based separatist notions. We have a million things in common and issues of healthcare represent the one big issue that we all share, regardless of rank or origin. If you cannot feel pain, you're not really human, in the true sense of being in full contact with the world around you. If we are connected only through the pain we bear then I want no part of this world; instead, I'd like to offer an idea that we can connect through our happiness as well. Happiness and sadness, pain and pleasure, rich or poor – it doesn't matter – we can share all. As long as we accept that we are part of the human race and that sharing makes us whole.

The commandment exists not because we want it to but simply because it has to. For reasons beyond the common collective understanding, life is not delivered in a flat, linear sequence with predictable outcomes. We are born and we die. In-between these two events, we must live. We want to live. We want the best from life, else we waste this life. We don't know what will happen next and we cannot undo what was done in the past. The only moment in which we ever had the chance to change, was the moment that passed just a second ago. This is how easily we miss the chance at affecting change. We realize sometimes that we missed it, but instead of making the change the very next moment, we spend exorbitant

146

amounts of energy in self-inflicted psychological warfare that sometimes last for years, in the odd case, a lifetime. After we're born, we grow. It's not our choice, we just grow. It has to be simply because it has to. After many cycles of growth we die (not all are fortunate enough to see those many cycles). The simplicity is, while we're living we seek the best of life. The best of life entails the best health, the best food, the best relationships, the best of anything, of everything. We are currently bound to the idea that economic wealth adds significantly to our quality of life, but in so many instances it had been made apparent that such is not the case. There is this sad, widely-believed construct that anything best is necessarily expensive. There are many of the richest people with the lowest quality of life and there are poorer people who live great lives. I bet that many of the latter is healthier that most of the former. We need to get unstuck from these ill-fated beliefs or constructs for they are hampering our progress to a lighter life, with more enjoyment and happiness. We'll continue to explore, travel, raise kids, make homes and overthrow governments, but to what extent do those things influence the quality of our lives? Tyrants have come and many of them are still active but we do not seem to realize that our dependence on their provisions placed them in power over us. Once we accept the responsibility to self, tyranny will neither be needed nor fueled. It would be a wasted life if one was to wait till the government becomes more "me-friendly" – what if it doesn't happen in your lifetime, as would be the case for many of the baby-boomer generation?

We are under political and economic control, even if we don't allow ourselves to outright admission of this fact, but we do not have to be as dependent on the public offerings as we believe we have to be. Being more independent does not mean you do not have to utilize what is offered, it simply means you have more of the choice to use it or not. As a community of people we can be more interdependent. Interdependence can allow communities to build solid platforms for health and happiness. The proactive approach would serve to build a foundation for health that could significantly minimize the chances of having to be forced into the situation of being dependent on expensive healthcare services in a later stage of life; we cannot stop one-hundred percent of diseases one-hundred percent of the time, but we can surely decrease the odds of being forced to accept an unhealthy lifestyle and a debilitating set of health outcomes when we are too old and too weak to build those foundations. Proactive means "before-action"; it is done to prevent things from happening *before* they have a chance to happen, hence the term preventative medicine, or preventative health. While you're young (i.e. *before* you're old) you build the foundation. Your parents are there to help you build while you're too young to stand or talk; when you reach the stage of conscientiousness you then help yourself or your prodigy to build. If you're old enough to read these lines of text or have them read to you, and you are able to understand these terms, then you're old enough to start taking the sense of responsibility for your own health. You do not have to be rich to be able to learn how to take responsibility for your own health.

Some of us do things with more conviction if we know things are sanctioned by a power higher than ourselves. The word commandment is commonly and mostly used for certain religious admonishments, but in the earlier days of the English language, people spake of commandments more frequently within everyday discourse (in the same, spake is the archaic past tense

148

form of speak). I purposefully named this chapter "Tenth Commandment", being fully aware of it potentially being linked to the biblical *Ten Commandments*. This book is not a religious treatment, but the idea is that the same manner of importance is attached to approaching the issue of health. The intended meaning of the word commandment, for the purposes of this book, and for use within *The New Dispensation of Health*, is a formal proposal to buy at a specified price, as in the noun bid (as at an auction). I am selling to you the idea of better, more satisfying personal health. Even more telling is the verb meaning of the word bid, namely making a serious effort to attain something. The election bid comes to mind, but right now I'm not running for political office. From the visual thesaurus (www.visualthesarus.com) the word bid is related to the much grander word beseech, which simply means to ask for or request earnestly. After reading the book and arriving at this point, the context of the Commandment of Health should be clear: you must invest in your health more seriously and I trust that you do not find this price too steep, for the consequences of not making such an investment is too dire even to mention! I beseech you – do not walk away without making this investment! In fact, the money to buy this book is negligible if you consider that applying a simple concept from it may bring generations of fortune and well-being, all of which cannot be measured in any amount of currency.

The commandment is made based on prior knowledge of a law that exists in nature, a law that manifests whenever we do not live in harmony with our surroundings. The Earth is not happy; she is violently moving air, water and land. The energies around her are unbalanced and she must find a new balance, a new equilibrium. We do not know how it will be and how much of it we will see, but what we can do right now is to accept that we can have the benefit of a more productive and progressive life. If we dare over-focus on the future, the present does not translate into any significant meaning, and even more sadly, the lessons of the past become entirely obsolete. We owe it to ourselves and those entrusted to us to take better care of ourselves and of our health. We can obey the individual-focused law of healing (page 34); it is reasonably achievable, not asking for more than a mere change of heart based on current, more updated knowledge. Procrastination is the enemy of proactivity; the former a vicious enemy, and if given a slight chance, The Procrastinator will bring with him the ominous dark clouds of more chronic suffering and despair; this we simply cannot allow.

~THE END of volume 2~

ACKNOWLEDGMENTS

I wish to acknowledge the following people:

- *L'amore della mia vita*, Tea De Santis – without whom this project would still just be a mere dream – whose design expertise and gentle hands are responsible for the artwork contained in this series. She continues to be an inspiration.
- Anu Garg and his efforts, through the beloved Word-of-the-Day feature as found at the URL www.wordsmith.org; it converts the serious, time-consuming act of writing into the sort of delightful play that brightens even the darkest corners of the undeveloped mind; such it does with an explosive luminescence worthy of contending the *Big Bang* in modern-day cosmology.

DISCLAIMER

This book was written with the intent of offering a reevaluation of certain deeply held concepts within our current modes of healthcare practice, be it philosophical or practical; no sentence has been written with the purposeful intent of injuring the reputations of any individual or organization. It is a personal statement more than an authoritative guide in the philosophy of contemporary healthcare, and mainly aims to draw interest for the sake of continuing a progressive discourse on matters of importance, whether on bases of public, political, socioeconomic or scholarly disciplines. If I do not fulfill these criteria, and I do manage to cause injury, I apologize, and shall do so in personal writing, if necessary. The future of healthcare services provision looks bleak, by all current indications; this volume has been written for purposes of setting a different mood within discussions pertaining to healthcare, and together with Volume 1, can be seen as the contribution of a lifetime by an independent researcher who witnessed the abysmal failures of many current systems in attempts to cater for the healthcare needs of growing populations in increasingly complex social environments.

Nathaniel W. Wilson

15 January 2014

"Unless someone like you cares a whole awful lot, nothing is going to get better. It's not."

Dr. Seuss

www.ingramcontent.com/pod-product-compliance
Lightning Source LLC
Chambersburg PA
CBHW040821180526

45159CB00001B/14